THE
NO COMPROMISE
BLACK
SKIN
CARE *Pro Edition*
GUIDE

THE SKIN
PROFESSIONAL'S CULTURALLY
INTELLIGENT TOOL FOR
CARING FOR DARKER
SKIN

BY C. R. COOPER

The Skin Theologian

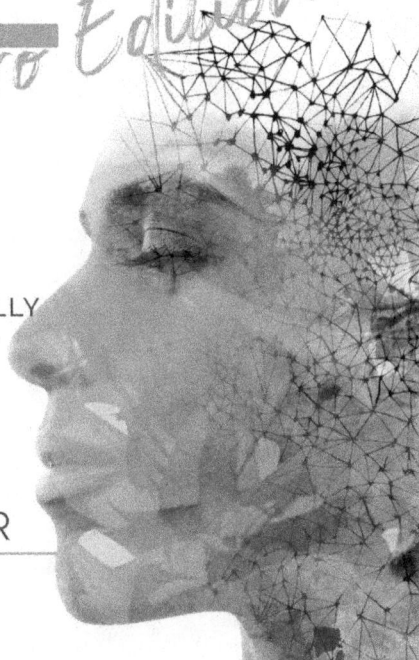

THE NO COMPROMISE BLACK SKIN CARE GUIDE "PRO EDITION"

THE SKIN PROFESSIONAL'S CULTURALLY INTELLIGENT TOOL FOR CARING FOR DARKER SKIN

C. R COOPER: THE SKIN THEOLOGIAN

www.skintheologian.com
IG: @THESKINTHEOLOGIAN

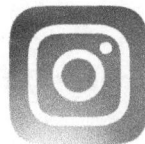

CONTENTS

Dedication

Thank you to all the readers and advocates of Volume 1 and of Skin Health Equity.

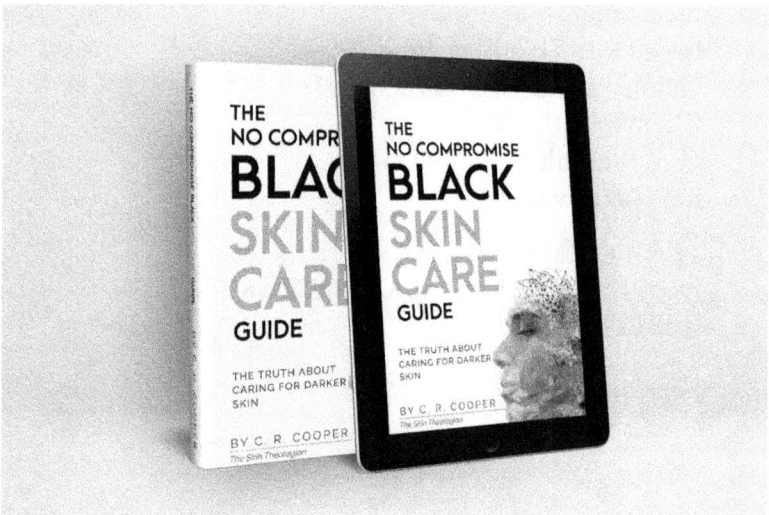

From every walk of life - ranging from seasoned pros through to new skin professionals and enthusiasts, your input was essential to the growth of greater advocacy around this topic.

You can still get your copy of Volume 1 here at IG @theskintheologian, if you haven't already picked up your copy.

This Pro Edition is dedicated to anyone who has felt an imbalance in resources available about darker skin concerns and/or who has ever struggled to confidently treat black skin as a professional.

Thank you for leveling up your knowledge, and for your courage to not shrink back.

We need more people like you in the industry

Special Note

This is by no means a textbook, but rather an invaluable and supportive resource for any Skin Professional (seasoned or new), who is passionate about continued growth in order to offer truly inclusive and Culturally Intelligent services within today's culturally awakened beauty industry.

I'd love to stay connected with you beyond this resource. I hope you will too.

— C.R.COOPER

Connect with me on IG at: @theskintheologian

and/or connect at www.skintheologian.com
for additional resources and updates.

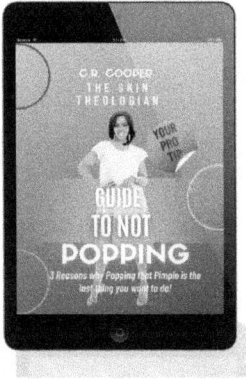

We have more work to do in advocating for greater Skin Health Equity. Thank you for joining me and so many others, one resource at a time.

Introduction

Despite being a billion-dollar industry, the global beauty industry still struggles with a lack of knowledge, awareness and information about darker skin tones.

This is improving, but the truth is that - despite black and brown skin tones being in the global majority - in the US, Canada and Europe the beauty industry has emphasized lighter skin.

If you think back to your childhood - were you ever truly told about taking care of your skin? Or did you have to learn through trial and error?

A big problem is that this "independent learning", without guidance, continues throughout life. Although we can all take responsibility for our own education and level up our skills, why is learning about dark skin never on the agenda?

Even as a skin care professional or health care professional, the information available is scant at best. Thankfully, this is getting a little better, but it still feels like there's a bit of a way to go yet.

For example, a high-profile analysis of dermatology textbooks have shown that as little as 4% to 18% of images contained within them show dark skin.

This type of study was first published in 2006. Here we are in the 2020's, and we're still looking at numbers under 20% when it comes to representation of common skin conditions in black skin.

Even in writing this book as a skin professional with significant experience and contacts around the world, sourcing imagery of skin conditions on darker skin tones has been a challenge. I've approached dermatologists, reviewed dermatology journals and discussed this with my peers. There are a number of projects taking place currently to bring skin health equity and representation up to date in research and educational resources, but this will take time to implement fully (unfortunately).

In my experience as a skin professional, and as a black woman, I have found finding images of people who look like me in dermatology textbooks to be challenging to say the least.

Even when I've approached dermatologists to ask for their help on this (thinking perhaps I haven't looked in the right places), they've admitted that these images aren't available. Most permitted images that they have access to are on lighter skin. How does that make sense?

I think that this is a sign of two things:

1. Skin conditions in darker skin are being missed because of a lack of awareness of what conditions look like and how they present themselves in black skin.
2. A lack of equity in the industry between dark skin and skin which is, quite frankly, completely unacceptable.

There are fewer dermatological studies on darker skin tones for professionals to learn from too. So even if pro's are ready to gain knowledge, they're going to have a harder time accessing the right information.

How's that for an example of skincare inequality?

This lack of representation means that beauty professionals leave their education unclear on how a myriad of skin conditions present themselves in darker skin and what the needs of black and brown skin actually are. This can lead to clients being excluded or receiving the wrong advice (and even damaging their skin).

As we covered in Volume 1, black dermatologists are in a minority (just 3% of US dermatologists are black). Of those who aren't black, 47% feel that their medical training doesn't prepare them to treat black skin.

Many skin care professionals don't feel empowered with the knowledge to work with black skin safely. There's a perception that it's "difficult" or needs to be handled with care. But let's be honest, that's true for *all* skin types, not just black skin. Would you want to go to a skincare professional who *wasn't* careful with your skin, whether your skin is dark, light or somewhere in between?

Exactly, me neither.

Every time a professional works on a client's skin, whatever tone, type or age that skin is, they should be handling it with care, addressing their concerns and working to meet their client's needs.

No gatekeeping. No "we can't treat your type of skin". No "I can recommend someone else for you". It's unnecessary.

Unfortunately it doesn't stop there either.

The majority of brands and publications assume that their customer or reader looks like them (and that is probably not black, based on the stats), and that's reflected in their marketing material, messaging, product development and product testing.

If there is a lack of diversity or representation on the teams that create these campaigns and make the decisions on how to market to skin professionals, consumers or create products and culturally-inclusive technologies, it probably never crosses their minds that they're missing something crucial. They're missing out on that experience and knowledge.

AI technology is starting to become more commonly used in the skincare and dermatology industry to identify, diagnose and treat skin. This technology is often programmed using algorithms based on light-skinned data, so routinely fails to recognise darker skin.

Education, empowerment and a sharing of resources is the only way that the industry will improve the way that it works with dark skin.

Clients shouldn't have to feel like they can't find someone who has the right knowledge, skills and experience - and is willing to work on their skin. Skincare is a big deal, and is very personal. Dark skin isn't a contraindication and shouldn't be treated as such.

We need to open up the conversation within the industry itself, as professionals, to ensure that every skincare professional feels comfortable, confident and ready to work with every type of skin out there.

WHO AM I?

C.R. Cooper - Skin Theologian

I'm a skincare professional with approximately 25 years of experience in the industry at the time of writing. I've worked as an Education Manager and Master Educator for a renowned global Skin Institute.

I've traveled internationally educating others on skincare and working with clients to achieve their skincare goals. I understand how deeply personal skincare is, and how important it is.

When it comes to skincare, skin conditions and skin concerns I've seen and heard pretty much everything. Including how many clients are frustrated that they can't find someone who understands their skin, and on the flip side, how many skincare professionals are stressed out at the thought of treating a client with dark skin. They don't feel confident or comfortable making recommendations or working with melanin-rich skin.

As a skincare professional and educator that's hard to hear.

I've also (quite literally) written the book on black skin care. In 2021 I published a book for enthusiasts and industry professionals alike, to help them learn more about caring for black skin and dispel all of the myths and misconceptions that are out there.

It's called **The No Compromise Black Skin Care Guide: The Truth About Caring For Darker Skin (Volume I)** and is available on Amazon. It's a great companion to this book, which is aimed, of course, at skincare professionals though the education within is available for all.

I also have a Master's of Divinity in Theology, which is where my expertise as your Skin Theologian comes in.

It helps with my holistic, empathetic approach to education.

I'll be sharing the things you need to know as a skin professional to ensure that you're able to confidently understand and treat your clients with darker skin.

If you will allow me, I would like to remind you that as a skin professional, it's your responsibility to ensure that you take the time to continue to educate yourself about the skin of your clients, and in turn educate them on the best way to take care of their skin. There are a lot of myths, misconceptions and rumors when it comes to the beauty industry. This is no different when it comes to black skin, and in fact, the unfamiliarity and lack of education around it is at the root of some of this confusion.

Let's level up our knowledge and level the playing field for our clients - every single one of them.

IT'S TIME TO TALK

2020 wasn't much fun for anyone. It was a sobering reminder for all of us of how quickly changes can be made, but also just how disconnected we can be from one another.

It offered an opportunity for industries and companies to measure their levels of equity centric or inequity-centric models of business.

During the summer of 2020, I was asked to join an *inclusivity board* for a major Beauty Association in Canada. The board consisted of skin and hair professionals of *every* ethnicity. Major brands, independent professionals and educators were at the (virtual, of course) table and met biweekly with efforts to assess and discuss what was going on in the world and how we needed to take the opportunity to drive change.

You could say that we were asked to form a coalition or "dream team" for normalizing inclusivity in every aspect of the industry. Hopefully you know by now, that this is everything to me. This point where I could see change taking place in an industry I've been so passionate about for such a long time.

We looked at the current deficiencies and realities of the beauty business with hopes to effect change. Some discussions were optimized by great collaborative thinking.

Other discussions were tethered to expressions of past disappointments, but ultimately, the common thread that brought every participant together, was the desire to make a difference.

As the meetings continued to progress, I began to realize that there were quite a lot of circular discussions without anything really being done.

This was something that we'd seen reflected in the media where some brands were keen to show their commitment, without actually doing the commitment part.

Back to the discussion. The circular feel to some of the conversations started to cause some frustration and uncertainty as to whether this approach was going to elicit change.

There were only a handful of skin professionals/educators (three of us, including me) on the board in comparison to the greater number of hair professionals/educators (I'd estimate 10-12) and a couple of marketing experts.

At the close of summer with the onset of fall and an uncertain continuing pandemic, the group ceased in its meetings (to my knowledge). All of that talk, momentum and discussion, but I wasn't sure what happened next.

It was at that moment, when I realized that I had a choice. I could write it off as weeks of wasted time, or I could see it for what it actually was: weeks of insightful conversation that demonstrated a need and desire for change.

I grew to realize that I, as a skin professional, had a responsibility to help to make a difference for greater equity, awareness and celebration of all ethnicities, especially of the ethnicities who have been underrepresented for years. In this case, those with black skin and darker skin.

And any effective change could only be accomplished through the mitigation of continued ignorance and fallacies around skin of color. That could only come from resources - educational resources at that.

I immediately searched online for resources that I could find that helped to level the education ground for darker skin. To my shock and disappointment, at the time, I couldn't find any that were not biased towards a skincare line or brand of technology.

There were no conversations being had in a wider context, without a product bent sales goal at the root of it. How disappointing for everyone who sought to learn more about skin of color, level up their knowledge and embed cultural intelligence and sensitivity into their skincare practice.

Remembering that I had a responsibility to make a difference where I could, I decided to create resources that could help all skin enthusiasts, and skin pros from all backgrounds, learn to celebrate and appreciate the wealth of diversity in the skin of color community. So here we are.

Since then, I am honored to know that I am not alone. There are many more who also share the same advocacy and are making differences in their spheres of influence.

So here's to a celebration of continued adequate education on darker skin. The Truth About Caring For Darker Skin!

The Skin Theologian.
(aka Char)

1

CREATING THE CULTURAL INTELLIGENCE (CQ) TREATMENT SPACE

*I*n this chapter, you'll learn about:

- What Cultural Intelligence (CQ) is and why it's important.
- How to feel comfortable and make sure your clients are comfortable when it comes to cultural conversations and interactions.
- Why leadership matters for CQ.

WHAT IS CULTURAL INTELLIGENCE?

Let's start out with a basic principle that underpins exactly what this book is about.

Cultural Intelligence (CQ) is the basic principle that underpins exactly what this book is about.

I was speaking on a skin panel of experts answering questions from clients, in our diversity skin discussion, when one virtual audience member asked a question. She asked "If I could recommend for her a Skin Professional who was black to treat her black skin."

Because we were discussing the myths to dispel about dark skin, I knew she felt confident that I would, without hesitation, refer someone to her that I had already vetted in my network of great skin professionals. My answer surprised her. I first assured her that research for the right skin professional was certainly needed but to not make the mistake of looking for someone who looked like her as a qualifier because that simply was an inaccurate way to find the right skin pro for her. What she wanted was an exceptional skin pro who was culturally competent when it came to treating clients.

These types of interaction will come into play every time you interact with someone else with a different background or culture to you - whether that's a client, a fellow beauty/skin health pro or someone else connected to your business.

That basic principle is this:

CULTURAL INTELLIGENCE

Cultural Intelligence (also known as CQ) is the ability to be able to relate and work effectively in culturally diverse situations. It's the ability to have cultural sensitivity and awareness in situations that are culturally diverse.

For some people, this comes naturally. For others, it's something that they learn in their interactions with others through experience.

It's not just an awareness of other cultures, it's the ability to interpret people's words and actions in line with their cultural communication styles. This allows for better communication, empathy and understanding.

All of those qualities are essential when you're working in a person-centered, touch-based industry like the beauty and skincare industry. You'll meet different people with different backgrounds and life experiences in your working life. It's important to be able to connect with the people around you.

I cannot emphasize enough how essential connection is in order to give your clients the best experience, grow your understanding of others, improve your communication skills and allow your business to grow.

SKIN THEOLOGIAN'S TIP

Take the time out to think about your clients and their cultural background.

Think about where your business is based and the local community. Is your customer base representative of the community? Is that community diverse?

Consider any **unconscious bias** you may have as a skincare professional - whether that's your perception of a client's behavior, how you interact with them or how to treat their skin.

How would you rank **your** own cultural intelligence?

There are no right or wrong answers here, but getting some perspective is usually a useful starting point.

Did you learn anything new about yourself or your behavior?

INCORPORATING CULTURAL INTELLIGENCE INTO YOUR TREATMENT SPACE

Unfortunately, many black clients have had negative experiences with the beauty industry over time.

Whether that's the struggle to find the right products, not enough representation, a lack of understanding of treatments and techniques that work for their skin or an experienced skin professional who's comfortable and confident in working with darker skin tones.

Let's be honest, this isn't acceptable.

First of all, let's talk about some terms that are often used interchangeably but aren't the same. The difference between them is important:

- **Culture** is a collection of behaviors and beliefs associated with a particular group.
- **Race** is a group of people related by common descent or heredity.
- **Ethnicity** is the identity with, or membership of, a particular racial, national or cultural group and observance of that group's customs, belief and language.

I think understanding these differences is an important part of framing the conversation around cultural intelligence and identity when it comes to clients and conversations.

Culture is, and can be, created by our beliefs and practices, bringing a quality to that environment that is made up of traditions, arts, education and training.

So essentially, our clients bring that culture when they enter a treatment space. The treatment space (and the business it sits in) also has a culture. As skin pro's our role is to contextualize that culture by establishing an environment that serves all cultural purposes and creates a cross-cultural environment.

Here's how you can incorporate more cultural intelligence into *your* treatment space as a professional, indifferent of your own personal ethnicity:

- Educate yourself on all skin tones, conditions and how they present themselves on a range of different types of skin.
- Learn about the key active ingredients that you should use for different types of skin and for darker skin tones. Not all active ingredients are as effective or safe for all skin.
- Be empathetic to all clients - even if you can't personally identify with a situation or concern, you can empathize with that person.
- Pay attention to your client and the small non-

verbal cues that they may give you as part of their cultural identity.

- Be respectful of culture and adapt treatments, products or routine if you need to do <u>this</u> (without compromising the skin's integrity).
- Practice tolerance and acceptance - things might be different to your personal experience and approach, but that's ok and is part of cultural intelligence.
- Help others to learn and ensure that any training or educational resources are inclusive and culturally aware.
- Adjust the way you interact with clients and colleagues to be culturally sensitive without being culturally fearful.
- Keep up to date with training and new industry information that relates to advances, breakthroughs and new studies.
- If in doubt, ask someone you trust and know well for advice or guidance on what you need to consider in your space. Remember to do this in a sensitive and culturally aware way with someone who is happy to discuss this with you - it isn't up to others to educate you, sometimes you need to learn first.

SKIN THEOLOGIAN'S TIP

Let's talk about trust.

Particularly in relation to my last point about asking someone that you know and trust for guidance if you aren't sure.

The trust and existing relationship is key here. If you have someone who is of a different culture to you, who you know is happy to talk about cultural issues and guide you to the best way to be sensitive to others, then that's wonderful.

However, if you ask someone - with the best of intentions - that you don't have that comfortable relationship with - for pointers on how to engage with people of their race or culture, it can come across as a little weird.

Speaking as a black woman, (rather than my role as an educator where you can ask me whatever you want, whenever you want), it can sometimes come across as insensitive when I'm expected to be an encyclopedia of blackness in every situation. Every black individual will have their own perspective and just because I'm ok with something, doesn't mean everyone else will feel the same.

Even within the black community, there's such a diverse experience of heritage, culture and environment. Being black certainly doesn't mean that we all have the same experiences or perspectives.

Be sensitive, careful and empathetic when you ask for guidance. Ask for this guidance from someone you know well, trust and have a close relationship with.

If they don't want to give you that guidance, then it's up to them. I hope that they would, but I understand why they might not.

LEADING BY EXAMPLE

If you're a beauty professional in a leadership role or a position of influence, setting a good example of cultural intelligence becomes even more important.

Also, let me take this opportunity to say: well done! The beauty, skincare and aesthetics industry is hugely competitive and your drive, dedication, determination and professionalism has helped you to rise to the next level.

You're a really important part of how we build cultural identity, understanding and awareness within the industry.

Without senior leaders, salon managers and educators who also embody the vision and values of cultural IQ (also known as CQ) then the ideas and work around it are lost.

You have the ability to shape the attitudes, beliefs and cultural awareness of the team around you.

First and foremost, being culturally competent is important for your clients and for the industry as a whole. But secondly: being culturally sensitive and understanding the needs of your clients is also *great for your business.*

Think about it. If you're turning a whole section of clients away because you "don't treat their skin tone" then that's a customer lost forever. It's income that will never set foot in your treatment space. It's repeat business that isn't ever going to be yours.

Their skin color isn't going to change, so if you've said no then they're going to find someone else who says yes. *You're* going to be the thing they change, not their skin.

Your attitude and approach *can* change.

There's also absolutely no way that the "turning paying customers away" (because let's be real, that's *exactly* what you're doing by being scared to work on black skin) makes sense as a business owner, sales lead or manager.

As a side note, black women spend around **nine times** more on hair and beauty than their lighter-skinned counterparts.

Now *imagine* you're turning away a customer who is going to spend nine times as much as a customer that you happily usher through the door for their treatment. You're going to have to find another eight clients from somewhere just to cover the difference (I know it's not that simple, but let's pretend it is for a sec).

Do you know how tough it can be to find - and *retain* - eight new clients and keep them all happy? Never mind keeping them booked into their regular slots in a way that fits into your working hours, treatment space opening hours and your availability.

I absolutely do. From the professionals I speak to and work with, It's hard work, stressful and the quickest route to burn out, irritated clients and a lackluster reputation.

Does that make business sense to you? It doesn't to me.

It's time to brush up on your CQ, educate yourself on the skin types of your clients (*all* of them) and make more money.

As a human, it should go deeper than just a business transaction and a demographic that spends more money on your services on average. But even if we strip it back to cold hard cash (or plastic or a digital transaction), business acumen and making as much money as you can: exclusion is out.

Inclusion will help your business to make more cash and keep your working life in check.

It also doesn't make sense from the perspective of someone who's risen to a leadership role in such a people-focused industry.

Unless those in a leadership role embody the values of CQ, they're just words that no-one really understands.

It's up to you to make it a priority and see it as something that your business lives by, rather than just another box to tick.

It's also important to empower your teams with CQ, create diverse teams with a range of different life and cultural experience and promote those who have that CQ within your business. It's a powerful skill to have, and other employers will snap that right up.

According to President and Partner at the Cultural Intelligence Center and author of *Leading with Cultural Intelligence: The Real Secret to Success*, David Livermore, it's been proven that the level of CQ amongst those in senior leadership is the most consistent variable linked to "whether or not an organization functions in the world with a track record of dignity and respect."

To embed CQ into the leadership in your organization, think about:

- Business goals and targets.
- Roadblocks or challenges that stop you from hitting those goals and targets.
- How culture plays a part in these challenges.
- How better CQ could help your team/organization to accomplish its goals and overcome challenges.
- Your hiring practices and representation.
- The attitudes, education and motivation of your teams when it comes to CQ.
- Asking the (right) questions, seeking opinions and finding out what you need to do when it comes to CQ.
- Taking it further than a half-day training session in diversity that leaves everyone feeling bored and disengaged. People need to be able to connect to make it feel right for them.

- When you carry out research, cite examples or work out your customer base - think about whether that's a diverse cultural representation or if it's one-dimensional.
- Measurement. It's not just a numbers game, but without any form of measurement, how do you know the impact of CQ in your team or treatment space?

Once you actually stop to think about CQ in this way, you'll find out just how important it is. To your business, your team, your clients and the world around you. CQ is you.

Another thing, CQ isn't just for your teams who have an "international" role, such as a lead skin pro, brand ambassador or educator. It's for every single person in your team. We live in an increasingly diverse, globalized world - staying in your lane isn't an option.

If this is you in a leadership role in the industry, I'm here to tell you: you've got this. You can make the change and encourage others to follow suit.

Lead by example and ensure that your team treats everyone with respect, kindness and the right knowledge, advice and guidance for their skin care and wellbeing needs.

AN IMPORTANT POINT ABOUT CULTURE

Part of CQ is understanding and accepting cultural differences, adapting to work within cultural boundaries, values and norms and valuing what other cultures have to offer.

It's not about 'othering' where people are made to feel like they don't fit in and that they sit outside of 'the norm'. It can also mean attributing negative characteristics to those people who are seen as the 'other' and removing their dignity.

Around the world, people with black and brown skin are regularly made to feel like an 'other', despite the fact that there are more people in the world who are not light skinned. This obviously changes depending on where you are in the world.

It isn't about stereotyping either. If you're not aware of what a stereotype is, it's where you have a fixed, over-simplified image or idea of a person, group of people or a tangible thing. It insinuates that every person who fits into a certain group is the same.

It *is* about equality. And about a skincare industry where everyone can have access to the same, effective treatments that's tailored to meet their needs. Where they can receive advice that's actually relevant to their skin, rather than being turned away and told that "sorry, we don't deal with your type of skin."

Skin *care* is really, really important - as is building up a skincare routine that's right for you and addresses any issues that you might have.

However, at the end of the day skin is skin.

The basics are the same whatever tone your skin is. The general order of the routine is the same, but with different ingredients, concentrations or concerns.

The fact of the matter is that skin care and treatments should *always* be adjusted to the individual's needs. If those needs include hyperpigmentation or avoiding certain acids that cause inflammation in darker skin then so be it.

Darker skin is *not* a contraindication to treatment and shouldn't be treated as such (much, *much* more on that in Chapter 2 - I've been ready for this conversation for a little while now).

While there are shared cultural experiences, cultural differences and situations that might need a different perspective, the most important things that you can do as a professional is to be understanding, be respectful and to be kind.

**"So Char, you're saying to treat everyone the
same but also treat them differently depending
on their culture? How do I even do that? I don't
know where to start."**

I often say "we can't truly celebrate or acknowledge
what distinguishes us until we learn to celebrate or
acknowledge what unites us." Think about it as being
about equality and skin health equity rather than
feeling like you're walking on eggshells. Treating
everyone respectfully and with kindness and understanding is the best starting point. Then tailoring your
interactions to make them feel comfortable, as you
would with any client, is the next step.

I get it, there's a fine line and it can feel complicated.
But it really isn't. For the most part, treating people like
the human-being they are is the fastest route to being
inclusive and culturally aware.

If you feel weird about saying something, or you aren't
sure if what you're about to say is offensive then it's
best to err on the side of caution. If you're saying something that fits into a stereotype of a group that someone
belongs to (that you don't), you probably shouldn't
say it.

A conversation that acknowledges darker skin and the professional context that you're in - treatment and product recommendations, skincare concerns, the fact that darker skin also needs SPF (again, more on that later) - is absolutely fine. The client is there for your professional advice and opinion.

It's only by being open, honest and respectful - along with the right education, skills and empowerment - that these conversations and approaches *will* get easier.

HOW TO HAVE A CULTURALLY INTELLIGENT CONVERSATION WITH YOUR CLIENTS

No-one wants to be canceled.

Most people don't want to make anyone feel uncomfortable or leave them feeling like they're an outsider.

It's partly because of this that people feel worried, awkward or afraid to have conversations that they feel might be seen as offensive. It comes from a good place.

Big spoiler alert: I'm going to let you in on a little secret...your black clients are *well* aware that they're black. It's not something that they're embarrassed to talk about, nor should they be, and it isn't news to them.

They're proud of their beautiful, melanin-rich skin and they want your professional advice and guidance to help them take care of it. They want advice and products that are tailored to their skin type and the needs of their skin.

Second spoiler alert: The word 'black' isn't offensive. It's ok to talk to your clients about the fact that they have dark skin and that they have different needs to other skin tones, and products they should stay away from.

Here are my tips for a culturally intelligent conversation with your clients:

- If you're uncomfortable, uneasy or nervous about a CQ conversation with a client, then that discomfort can probably be felt by the client. Take small steps first and as you grow in confidence, you can continue to develop your CQ.
- Don't make assumptions.
- Ask questions where you need to, and don't be afraid to get more information where it's relevant to treatment or product recommendations.
- You're the expert when it comes to skin care,

but you may not be the expert in another person's culture. Be sensitive to their needs.

- Never make your client feel uncomfortable or like they're an outsider. No-one wants to feel like they're being "othered" or judged.
- Take the time to educate yourself about different types of skin and the ingredients that work best for them (and what should be avoided).
- Be sensitive and empathetic in the way you speak and the words you choose. Think carefully about the language that you use, how it could be interpreted and speak confidently.
- Steer clear of any myths or misconceptions around black skin and darker skin tones - yes, all skin tones need SPF. No, not all black skin is oily. Yes, black *does* crack if the skin isn't taken care of.
- If you don't know the answer to a specific question - don't guess at the answer, but don't leave the conversation at a dead end. If you need to check, be honest about that and follow up.

Most of this is common sense and common courtesy with a big side order of professionalism. You've absolutely got this.

You don't need to have the same skin type or skin tone as your clients to be able to treat their skin and address their needs effectively.

Every client that walks through your door will not have the exact same type of skin, beliefs or experiences as you do. And that's a good thing - a great thing even - as it helps us to learn new skills and gain that all-important CQ.

BEING AN ALLY IN A PROFESSIONAL CONTEXT

Hopefully, you've heard of the term "ally" in relation to supporting black partners, friends, clients and colleagues.

In case you're not aware, to be an ally means to be someone who isn't part of an underrepresented group but takes action to support those who *are* part of an underrepresented group.

This is something that you can do in a professional context when you're working with colleagues and clients. It's important to help empower underrepresented groups and make changes that will help others to be seen, heard and successful.

An ally understands that, unfortunately, the scales aren't always evenly balanced in the workplace and takes a supportive role to help redress that balance.

Here's how you can be an ally to your colleagues and clients as a skincare professional:

- **Acknowledge Knowledge** - talk about the expertise you see from others, especially where promotions and performance is being discussed.
- **Dispel Stereotypes** - disengage or educate when you hear harmful stereotypes or negative discussion of others based on culture.
- **Ask Questions** - if your workplace isn't actively diverse or culturally intelligent, then ask why.
- **Advocate**- make sure that people are represented and invited to key meetings and events.
- **Educate** - educate yourself so that you can educate others in turn.
- **Speak Up** - it can be intimidating if you're in a cultural minority. As an ally, speak up if you see or hear things that don't sit well from a cultural perspective.
- **Support Others** - provide a listening ear and a

supportive, non-judgemental environment for others to share.

Being an ally takes courage and conviction, as well as the ability to put yourself in someone else's shoes and speak up, even when you aren't directly affected by something.

Ally support is an important part of CQ, diversity and inclusion. It's not about speaking on behalf of others, but instead supporting and empowering people to have their voice heard.

KEY TAKEAWAYS

- Education is essential for CQ and skincare equity.
- The ability to communicate effectively and professionally with a variety of clients *will* benefit your business and your own personal development.
- We need leaders who will embed CQ throughout their business and empower their teams to act with CQ and integrity.
- Allyship is important to build culturally intelligent spaces.

DARKER SKIN IS NOT A CONTRAINDICATION

*I*n this chapter, you'll learn about:

- The truth about those common misconceptions you hear when professionally treating black skin - including those advanced treatments.
- The benefits of seeing a skincare professional (that's you!).
- What treatments *are* actually a contraindication for darker skin.

GETTING TO THE TRUTH

Moving on from trust and cultural intelligence, it's time to talk about the opposite - those myths about black skin that play a big part in the confusion, concern and discomfort around treating your clients.

I'm going to jump right in with some of the most common misconceptions you might have heard as a skin pro when it comes to black skin.

Hands up if you've ever heard, believed or even repeated (to a client or a fellow skin pro) any of the following:

Black skin doesn't age.

While some parts of the media - and even the black community - will swear that we're all some sort of age-defying vampire who will continue to look 20 years old at the age of 90, the fact is….everyone ages.

The truth about black skin? Of course black skin ages! Whilst signs of aging may show up a little slower than those with lighter skin, they'll show up as you get older.

I think it's partly an unfamiliarity with darker skin that makes this misconception so popular. If you're not familiar with what a 40-year old black woman looks like, then it's easier to feel confused about age. Does that make sense?

I also think that the rise of treatments like wrinkle-freezing shots and filler along with more intense anti-aging skincare routines, plays a little part in this. Plus timelines are a little more fluid now. Some people look, act and feel older at 30, some people are 75 and act 'like a 30-year-old'. There are no set timelines.

Aging; it's a normal part of life that should be celebrated. Your life experience will show up on your face at some point. It's not a negative, and it isn't something to be worried about. It happens to everyone. It's not always about aspiring to look 25.

Black Skin Doesn't Need Sun Protection.

I'm just going to jump right in with the truth on this one. Black skin needs sun protection. Daily. Sunscreen and SPF needs to be part of a skin care routine **for everyone**. It's as essential as cleansing.

While it's true that black and brown skin contains more melanin (and therefore slightly more natural protection) than lighter skin, it's by no means immune to sun damage and the consequences of it.

People with darker skin can still get sunburnt (but you may not recognize it as sunburn as easily as on lighter skin), and that causes inflammation which is bad news for things like hyperpigmentation and scarring - as well as the fact that sunburn *hurts*.

This isn't just a misconception that non-black professionals believe either. Many, many people in the black community believe that they can't burn in the sun, or that they're immune to skin cancer. This is not the case and if - as a professional - you spot anything on your client's skin that you think looks suspicious or in need of medical attention, you must flag it.

Sunlight can be great for your health, as your body needs vitamin D. However, sun exposure can lead to premature aging, skin cancer, hyperpigmentation and melasma in all skin tones - including melanin-rich darker skin.

Let's jump to a little more detail about sunscreen. There are two different types of sunscreen that stop sun damage:

- **Physical (mineral) sunscreen** - ingredients like *Titanium Dioxide* and *Zinc Oxide* block the sun and scatter the rays before they penetrate your skin.
- **Chemical sunscreen** - ingredients like *Avobenzone* and *Octisalate* absorb UV rays before they damage your skin.
- A common complaint I hear from my black clients is that their sunscreen leaves a white cast on their skin that makes their skin look gray or ashy. If you hear this from your clients, ask them to try a chemical sunscreen

instead (there are some great brands out there).

Physical sunscreen uses ingredients like *Zinc Oxide* to block out the sun's rays, which is what leaves the white film behind that we all hate. Chemical sunscreens work differently and many formulations are clear when applied.

It's a sad truth but skin cancer is more likely to be diagnosed at a later stage in darker skin, which usually means it's more serious. It also means that melanoma survival rates are far lower - a 2019 CDC study found that the 5-year survival rate for melanoma was 66% for black patients compared to 90% for white patients. We'll touch on a specific form of melanoma that's more common in black skin in a bit. Yes, that's right, more common in black skin.

Black Skin Is Thicker Than Other Skin Types.

I hate this one. It's been a common misconception for far too long that black skin is stronger or doesn't feel pain the same way as other skin tones. Read that again. Does it not sound completely crazy to you that anyone would think that?

While black skin has more corneocyte layers and a more compact stratum corneum, which in theory equals 'stronger' skin when it comes to chemical and mechanical interactions, to think of all black skin as super-strong, extra-thick and able to take any sort of damage is dangerous.

In my experience as a professional, black skin can actually be *more* prone to damage and can show the effects of damage more easily (and for longer). It can be more prone to inflammation, hyperpigmentation and scarring than other skin tones.

Being rough or heavy-handed with any client's skin is a bad idea. You know that (I hope). I know that. So why would you think that's different for dark skin? Treat every client's skin in line with their individual needs and treat every client kindly.

Black Skin Is Always Oily.

People of all skin tones can have different skin types. Please, please don't assume that your black clients automatically have oily skin. This isn't true. Your black clients could have dry, combination or dehydrated skin (as well as oily). Just like everyone else.

You should be using your professional expertise and skills to correctly assess your client's skin type. Even if they think they have oily skin, or they've been told they have oily skin in the past - take the time out to actually work it out for yourself (and for your client).

Using the wrong products, ingredients and wrong treatments on your clients is bad news and could be terrible for their skin.

Black Skin Needs a Completely Specialist Routine From Start To Finish.

Again, I think this comes from unfamiliarity with working on dark skin and the misconception that it's completely different to lighter skin. In far too many cases, black skin is almost treated as a separate 'skin type' (alongside dry, combination, oily and sensitive skin types). Your routine should work with your skin type.

Black is not a dermatologically recognized 'skin type' in the way that dry or oily skin is. There are no products that I'm aware of that have been formulated for a 'black skin type' because that type doesn't exist. Black skin - just like every other skin type - can be dry, oily, combination, sensitive, dehydrated, congested, acne-prone.

It's impossible to take the viewpoint that black skin is a type and every single person with dark skin has the exact same skin and needs. Just look at the range of heritage, tones and locations throughout the world that the black community are in.

It's absolutely 100% true that some skincare ingredients and products should be avoided when working with black skin (*way* more on that later). It's also absolutely, 100% true that you **don't** need to rush out and buy an entire separate range of products that you only use on your dark skinned clients.

The way that some brands market themselves will also have you feeling confused by this. While there might be a cultural understanding of black skin and the needs of darker skin from some brands, that maybe isn't understood in more mainstream brands, this doesn't actually mean that their products work differently.

On the flip side, some brands market themselves to black consumers in a way that might make you think it's black-owned, but when you dig a little deeper it's not. It's just marketing. It's completely confusing.

If you support black-owned brands, I am absolutely all for that. But make sure that the products you use are right for your clients. Black-owned doesn't automatically mean "absolutely suitable for every black client that ever existed" and it's short-sighted on all sides to think that that's the case.

Only A Black Skin Pro Should Work On Black Skin.

This one probably stems from people being let down by a previous skin pro who didn't know how to work with their skin. Remember the woman I referenced earlier in the book who asked for my black skin pro recommendation, simply because she was black? They felt safer with a black skin pro who 'knew what they were doing'.

I've met amazing skincare professionals from every background. I've met some not-so-amazing skincare professionals from all walks of life (unfortunately).

The things that actually matter - far, far more than their skin color - is their education and expertise, professionalism, skills, product quality and that all-important cultural intelligence.

Black Don't Crack!

I hear this all the time! And like my previous point around aging. Black can crack, especially if a client isn't taking care of their skin. It might "crack" a little differently to other skin tones, but it certainly isn't invincible.

Dark Marks Are There Forever.

Dark marks, hyperpigmentation, dark spots - whatever you want to call them - are normal for skin of every color. They don't need to be there for the long term, there are plenty of simple, effective routines that will help to minimize the appearance of dark spots and hyperpigmentation safely.

Skin Bleaching Is Normal.

I wish you could see my face as I just typed the title of this paragraph. Skin bleaching should *never* be considered normal. Putting a corrosive substance on your face that leaves it susceptible to pain, damage and future health problems *isn't* normal.

Even products that are regularly touted as 'safe' for lightening dark marks (looking at you, **Hydroquinone**) should be avoided where possible and handled with care if avoiding isn't an option.

In some cultures within the black community, unfortunately 'lighter' is seen as better, which is what leads to people risking their health and skin in this way.

I'm going to tell you more about the dangers of skin bleaching, and how to have those conversations with your clients who you suspect might be lightening and damaging their skin later on in this book.

Black Clients Should Skip Laser Treatments and Skin Peels.

We're going to call this a partial truth for the time being. It's not a one-size-fits-all situation and while some laser treatments and chemical peels aren't suitable for darker skin, there are some alternatives that are more suitable.

We'll talk about that more in the laser drama chapter, because, well it is a little bit of a saga to be honest.

Acids Are Bad For Dark Skin.

This one is kind of partially true. Some acids are better than others for darker skin as they're gentler and cause less inflammation. Skin damage and inflammation can cause hyperpigmentation, which is a common concern in dark skin.

Prevention is better than handling hyperpigmentation once it's set in but there are solutions once you see signs of hyperpigmentation on the skin.

Dark Skin Doesn't Get Conditions Like Rosacea.

Just not true. While it may be less likely, it can happen. Back to the point about dermatology textbooks that don't show images of common skin conditions on black and brown skin - because people are less familiar with what it looks like it can get missed.

Rosacea is sometimes mistaken for acne in dark skin, because the redness usually associated with rosacea on lighter skin isn't always as visible. This can lead to incorrect treatment which can actually cause far more problems.

Treatments Like Anti-Aging Injections Aren't For Black Skin.

While there's still a little stigma around use of treatments like Botox and fillers in the black community, this is steadily on the rise. According to the American Society of Plastic Surgeons, around 11% of cosmetic procedures and 4% of Botox injections were carried out on black patients in 2020.

However, like many other treatments, the clinical studies of these treatments have almost exclusively been on lighter skin. Most of the media and marketing around these treatments doesn't show dark skin tones.

These treatments tend to be used slightly differently too. Lines and wrinkles can present themselves differently on darker skin tones compared to lighter skin tones - for example vertical lines between the eyebrows (commonly treated with Botox) are less common in black skin than in light skin.

As with any procedure that pierces the skin, clients need to choose and trust us because we are qualified practitioners who are experts at what we do. Scarring from poor injection technique or practice can lead to hyperpigmentation or keloid scarring if a practitioner isn't careful or experienced.

DON'T BELIEVE EVERYTHING YOU HEAR

Hopefully this clears up some of the misconceptions you may have had when it comes to treating black skin. So many of these myths have been repeated for so long that they just become something that people automatically believe to be true.

That then becomes a cycle of incorrect information which leads to poor or ineffective treatments and mistrust from the client. It's a vicious cycle that needs to be broken.

It's no wonder that these misconceptions, myths and misunderstandings have led to misinformation thriving for both clients and skin pros. This is why education and understanding is so important.

Seek out the education and truth that you - and your clients - deserve, so that you can ensure that you provide the best, safest and most effective treatment that you can.

INDUSTRY - REAL TALK

Let's talk about the beauty industry, and in particular the skincare industry. As a skincare professional you'll probably already know a lot of this stuff but it's always useful to recap and take a new perspective.

It's easy for people outside of the industry to write it off as something that's unnecessary or unimportant. They think the industry is just about "looking pretty", and that there's nothing more to it than that. Wow, are they wrong!

I realize I've started this chapter by talking about some of the misconceptions and the things that people get wrong about the black community. Well, this is going to take a closer look at the industry, the opportunities that are there and some of the things that people get wrong (and right).

WHERE ARE THE STATS AT?

Let's talk facts. Beauty and skincare industry facts to be more precise.

This will help us to see where we're at and provide the perfect springboard to talk about the industry in a little more detail. The good, the bad and the ugly.

The last few years haven't been easy for beauty pros across the world. There have been salon closures, increased costs of personal protective equipment, increased shipping delays, increased shipping expenses and clients who have cut down their salon visits over concerns about health.

Some clients have had no choice but to cut back because of changes to their budget as a result, even if they'd love to take up their treatments again.

The good news is that the extra time at home, the lack of distractions and - let's be honest - probably all of that extra time we *all* spent looking at our faces on Zoom has meant there's a renewed interest in skincare.

Let's look at some numbers that highlight just how important, and how much of a big deal, the beauty industry actually is.

CHART A

The Salon and Spa Market

01

It's estimated that the global salon and spa market will be worth $217.25 billion by 2026

02

The average beauty treatment spend in the US is $44 per person per year.

03

Millennials and Gen X spend the most on beauty treatments in the US - $51 a year on average over 9 treatments

04

Facials are the 6th most popular treatment for US women - 32% of women have a regular facial

05

Facials are the 3rd most popular treatment for men in the US - 26% of men have a regular facial.

The Beauty and Skincare Industry
The global beauty industry worth 2021: $511 billion 2025: $716.6 billion (estimated)
The Asia Pacific region holds 46% of the worldwide beauty industry market share
Skincare purchases make up 42% of the global beauty market
The global skincare industry growth is around 6% each year: 2012: $127.9 billion 2021: $148.3 billion 2025: $177.4 billion (estimated)
On average women spend up to $3,756 on beauty products each year

The Salon and Spa Market
(Seen in Chart A)
It's estimated that the global salon and spa market will be worth $217.25 billion by 2026
The average beauty treatment spend is $44 per person per year
Millennials and Gen X spend the most on beauty treatments - $51 a year on average over 9 treatments
Facials are the 6th most popular treatment for women - 32% of women have a regular facial
Facials are the 3rd most popular treatment for men - 26% of men have a regular facial
Beauty advertising spend is predicted to reach $7.7 billion in 2022
96% of beauty brands are on social media, with 82% of women believing that this is what dictates beauty trends

Those are some pretty impressive statistics that show just how valuable what we do is and where we make a difference.

One thing I would say is that I think average spends and salon visits are much higher - these stats will take into account people that don't visit the salon, and probably skew the figures a little. In my experience, those loyal clients who see a salon visit as an important part of their routine to look and feel great will visit a lot more regularly and value those services.

WHY OUR INDUSTRY IS SO IMPORTANT

The benefits of the beauty industry, being a skin professional and working with clients are huge. We're trusted advisors, confidantes, confidence boosters and educated professionals who make a difference to the lives of our clients.

For many, many people beauty goes much further than just skin deep, it's an important part of their self care routine.

Here are some of the things that I personally *love* about being a skincare professional:

- Helping clients to gain confidence and self-esteem by working with them to address issues they're having with their skin.
- Making a difference to the mental and physical wellbeing of clients.
- Being at the forefront of technological and scientific innovation.

- Getting to know clients on a personal level and seeing them open up (I love this one!).
- Making a difference to a client's life.
- Educating clients about their skin.
- Educating others in the industry about professional topics.
- Connection with other beauty pros.
- Being able to pick up on something that might need medical attention - you could quite literally save someone's life.
- The fact that the industry as a whole is extremely accessible.
- That it empowers and provides to women (and men, of course) across the world.

And here are some of things that aren't so great in the industry (you can probably guess some of them without me even writing them):

- The misinformation and misconceptions that fill the industry, leading to clients feeling frustrated and unheard.
- An occasional lack of transparency across the industry.
- The people who give advice as if it's fact, without having the right knowledge or information to share that knowledge.

- The brands and people in the industry who'll say or do pretty much anything if it means selling a product (I realize this isn't specific to the industry).
- That sometimes things feel inconsistent. Standards vary from place to place, legal frameworks are vague and information is unclear.
- Sometimes things get a little gimmicky. They focus on what's hot and what's not, rather than what's important.

That about sums it up for me - in short, the positives outweigh the negatives. A lot of the negative parts could be solved with the right education, training and knowledge sharing with consumers and pros alike.

How many of these positives and negatives do you agree with? Are there any others that you've experienced that stand out for you?

THE LIPSTICK EFFECT

In this context, I have to talk about the lipstick effect too as it goes to show just how people value their beauty routine and the things that make them feel good.

In short, the Lipstick Effect is where consumers still spend money on smaller, accessible indulgences at times of economic uncertainty. Times might be too tight for a new car, an exotic holiday and a whole new wardrobe, but they can probably afford a beauty product such as a lipstick. Hence the name, the Lipstick Effect.

For this reason, the beauty industry does tend to be pretty resilient, especially on the consumer side of things. People want to give themselves a boost, a distraction and a small luxurious treat, whatever else is going on. Beauty helps them to do just that without blowing their budget.

In fact, sales of small luxury items can actually be used as an indicator of an economic recession. Other items don't see this type of response when times are hard. But beauty does.

Another theory is that people make more of an effort to find work in an economic recession and as the labor markets become more competitive, people seek to look more professional and put-together for their interviews. Hence, they spend on beauty products.

It's worth noting that in times of severe economic difficulty, people will stop spending on extras entirely. Everything from coffee through to lipstick and everything else. During the pandemic however, we actually saw beauty sales soar as new brands entered the market and people took the time out to build up new routines.

Big caveat here: I'm not an economist, so if you want to learn more about predicting economic trends you may need to pick up a slightly different book to this one. But nevertheless, it's reassuring to know that you're part of a resilient industry.

WHAT DO THE SKIN PROS THINK ABOUT WORKING WITH BLACK SKIN?

We've talked about the industry in general - the good *and* the bad parts - so let's bring it back to the topic at hand.

What do the industry professionals really think about working with clients with darker skin tones from a professional perspective?

How comfortable do they feel in their practical knowledge of the needs of black skin? Where do they feel the gaps in their knowledge are?

If you read the last book - Volume I) (if you didn't, it's worth picking up I promise), you'll remember that I asked a lot of questions from skin professionals that I've known and worked with over the years on how confident they were in working with clients with dark skin. Absolutely no judgment, everything anonymous and everyone who I asked was encouraged to be as honest as they needed to be. I would have no idea who had answered what.

These skin professionals were in different locations around the world, at different points in their career and their experience of working with a culturally diverse range of clients was varied. Some of them worked for brands, some taught skin professionals in institutes, some were self-employed and some worked in skin centers, getting hands-on experience with clients.

The results were an eye opener and cemented just why things need to get better in the industry. I knew that things were falling short of where they needed to be but it was somewhat frustrating to see how far behind.

It highlighted the need for skin health equity and education for professionals across the industry.

When I came to write the book you're reading now, I decided to do another industry-specific survey. This time with a whole host of different beauty professionals.

I was hopeful that things were on the up and that there would be demonstrable progress.

Recognition of the different needs of black and brown skin along with recognition of the need for more education around these skin tones definitely seems to be on the rise. And that's just in the time between writing my first book and this one.

I'll reveal the findings from round two of the survey in a second, but first of all let's take a look at some of the progress that's been made in the professional beauty industry in just a short amount of time as the need for equality moves into the forefront.

- UK Hair and Beauty awarding body Vocational Training Charitable Trust (VTCT) made working with black skin and hair a part of their curriculum. Some US states, such as Louisiana, are bringing the same requirements into education in 2022. As I've said before, education is essential and opting out of certain lessons shouldn't be an option.
- Projects are taking place across the medical and dermatology industry to ensure that there's representation of how skin conditions present themselves on darker skin tones in text books and medical resources.
- There has been more representation of different ethnicities in advertising campaigns across the industry (whether it goes further

than that does remain to be seen in my opinion).

- Beauty brands have taken an inward look at what their internal teams look like and whether there's actual representation there through the #PullUpOrShutUp movement on social media. Many brands found themselves lacking under scrutiny and vowed to do better. This representation will be a good thing for innovation, understanding and education.

- There have been a whole host of new beauty brands that focus on black consumers at their core and the needs of black hair, skin and cultural considerations. This includes the basics like foundation shade ranges right through to specialist products for hair becoming way more than something you buy at a specific retailer or on a tiny corner of shelf in a mainstream one.

- Beauty brands, social media platforms and the advertising industry are working with more black creatives to showcase their skills and learn from their experience.

- Some beauty and education brands have stepped up to increase their diversity and wealth of knowledge, others have supported black causes to raise awareness, make more conscious inclusion choices and make donations.

- Product names and shade names are under more scrutiny to stop cultural appropriation and stereotyping. Some huge brands have removed names that focus on lighter skin as the goal - but it's worth mentioning that these products (usually aimed at lightening or brightening the skin in some way) still exist, they're just not called "fair", "white" or "lightening".

- More consumers are calling brands out where there isn't representation and inclusion. This is important because it affects brands publicly and in their purses, which unfortunately is sometimes the only way to elicit change.

- There's been more scrutiny of brands that are marketed to black consumers, to see if there actually is that representation at all levels.

- Social media site Pinterest introduced the ability to filter image searches of makeup, beauty products, hair care and skincare looks by skin tone and hair type, allowing people to curate their feed and find images, products and inspiration that's representative of them.

Again, some positive progress that's been made in a short amount of time. There's still a little way to go and things are far from perfect but positive changes are being made all of the time.

A lot of these negative situations have existed for far too long, they won't be unpicked overnight (unfortunately).

SURVEY RESULTS

I asked skin professionals within my network about their opinions on how they work with a range of different skin tones and photo-types. These contacts range from beauty brand founders, employees, practicing skin professionals and experts from around the world.

I wanted to get their professional perspective on a range of equipment, technology and training issues to discover just how they feel about the tools they have in the industry when it comes to all skin. I have to say, I found some of the results pretty refreshing.

Here's what I asked, and how these industry professionals responded. To view the visual info-graph, please see Chart B.

1. As a skin professional, do you have a particular piece of advanced technology that you feel is a 'must-have' for effective client treatments?

85% of respondents said yes, they regularly use advanced technology when they're working with their clients. They use it to get the best results in the treatments they carry out.

2. In your opinion is this piece of technology or equipment cross-cultural for all photo types?

92% said that yes, their favorite advanced piece of technology they used with clients worked for all skin types and tones. Unfortunately, this still means that 7% aren't able to treat all of their clients as effectively.

3. Were you trained on the Fitzpatrick scale, or any other type of photo measuring scale (at school level)?

Ok. Wow. Only 23% of respondents were trained to recognize and understand different skin tones. That means 65% have never received basic education on skin tones to underpin the rest of their training, and to understand the impact. A further 12% said that it wasn't necessary to learn this. Interesting.

While there will be some contextualisation to this (age, area of training, memory) this is a lot lower than I expected. The Fitzpatrick scale is not perfect by any means (I have a lot to say about this later on in the book) but it is *something* that adds a framework to skin tones and photo-types at least.

The worry with this is that skin tone and how to work with dark skin has never been discussed at a basic level to provide a foundation for the rest of their work. It's a basic that should be taken into consideration from the beginning of training right through to the later portion of an industry career. This training and knowledge is improving from what I can see, and I would hope that these professionals have taken the time to level up during their professional career.

I want to know more about the 12% who didn't feel that it's necessary to know about this! Maybe it's specific to their career niche, client base or their own additional training. I hope it's not an indication that they don't need to know this information, and that they'll be completely fine.

4. Were you trained on the Fitzpatrick scale when it came to determining thermal or light emitting energy tolerances?

77% of respondents said that they were, in fact, trained to use the Fitzpatrick scale when it came to thermal or light emitting treatments (laser, IPL etc). I'll go into more detail later in the chapter about why this isn't ideal, and my issues with the Fitzpatrick scale as a measurement method, but I will say that I wonder what the remaining 13% are using. I hope that it's something even more effective than Fitzpatrick, and I really hope that it doesn't mean that they were never actually trained to take skin tone into consideration when it comes to certain types of treatment. It's an *extremely* important thing to consider with these types of treatment.

5. Were you adequately trained or advised on the recovery protocol for photo or thermal damaged skin?

31% of respondents said that they'd received adequate training on the recovery period for this type of damage. This leaves 69% unaware of how to advise on recovery for this type of damage. What does this mean for clients that come looking for a solution to their skin damage? Further damage? This needs to improve.

6. Do you have, or are you aware of other unbiased technology that's available for skin professionals to use on all skin photo-types?

The answers went like this:

- Yes - 42%
- No - 42%
- Not necessary - 16%

The first thing that jumped out at me was the higher-than-expected percentage of 'not necessary' responses. I wonder why they think it isn't necessary? I hope that it's because they either have the professional expertise and experience to use this treatment on all skin tones. Or I hope it's because they have all of the inclusive, unbiased technology they need and their clients are happy with their treatments. I really hope that it isn't because every tone of skin should be treated exactly the same.

It's interesting too that the results of 'yes' and 'no' answers are spread 50/50. This shows some gaps in awareness or skin health equity to me.

7. Do you believe that education and training is as prevalent for unbiased technology as for other types of technology?

With this question, I wanted to try and get to the bottom of whether or not there's less training on unbiased technology (for a cross-cultured demographic - i.e. technology that's suitable for all photo-types and situations).

The answers went like this:

- Yes - 38%
- No - 54%

- Not necessary - 8%

So it was overwhelmingly felt that there wasn't relevant training on non-biased technologies vs technology that's only suited for certain skin. This is a true, visible example of a lack of skin health equity within the industry.

8. Have you seen or been aware of improper use of any technology where clients' skin has been damaged?

92% of skin professionals answered yes. This doesn't surprise me, as an educator and a skin care professional. It doesn't, however, make me any less disappointed. That's a huge amount of clients out there who have had their skin damaged by inexperienced, uneducated or unaware 'industry professionals'. That's damaging to the reputation of the entire industry - those clients are far less likely to recommend a product or service that's damaged their skin.

Some of this damage will have been permanent and irreversible. Some of it will have had an impact on confidence and self esteem. Some of it will have taken a significant amount of time and money to actually resolve. This is really, really sad - the thing that's even sadder is that I doubt anyone in the industry is surprised.

9. Do "more at risk" photo-types affect your confidence and choice of technology when it comes to your skin practice?

This was a relatively even split. 46% said that it did affect their confidence and choice of technology. 54% said that this didn't have an impact on their choices and confidence.

10. Do you believe that there are readily available technologies for the skin professional that aligns with a multicultural/cross-cultural clientele demographic?

A completely even split on this one. 50/50. So whichever way you look at it, half of the skin professionals surveyed aren't getting their needs met when it comes to multicultural and cross-cultural clientele. The result of this is a whole host of clients who will also not be having their needs met. Surely this isn't acceptable in the industry?

CHART B

Skin Professional's Survey Results

Q: 01
As a skin professional, do you have a particular piece of advanced technology that you feel is a 'must-have' for effective client treatments?

85% of respondents said yes, they regularly use advanced technology when they're working with their clients. They use it to get the best results in the treatments they carry out.

Q: 02
In your opinion is this piece of technology or equipment cross-cultural for all photo types?

92% said that yes, their favorite advanced piece of technology they used with clients worked for all skin types and tones. Unfortunately, this still means that 7% aren't able to treat all of their clients as effectively.

Q: 03
Were you trained on the Fitzpatrick scale, or any other type of photo measuring scale (at school level)?

Ok. Wow. Only 23% of respondents were trained to recognize and understand different skin tones. That means 65% have never received basic education on skin tones to underpin the rest of their training, and to understand the impact. A further 12% said that it wasn't necessary to learn this. Interesting.

Q: 04
Were you trained on the Fitzpatrick scale when it came to determining thermal or light emitting energy tolerances?

77% of respondents said that they were, in fact, trained to use the Fitzpatrick scale when it came to thermal or light emitting treatments (laser, IPL etc). I'll go into more detail later in the chapter about why this isn't ideal, and my issues with the Fitzpatrick scale as a measurement method, but I will say that I wonder what the remaining 13% are using.

Q: 05
Were you adequately trained or advised on the recovery protocol for photo or thermal damaged skin?

31% of respondents said that they'd received adequate training on the recovery period for this type of damage. This leaves 69% unaware of how to advise on recovery for this type of damage.

Q: 06
Do you have, or are you aware of other unbiased technology that's available for skin professionals to use on all skin photo-types?

The answers went like this:

Yes - 42% •
No - 42% •
Not necessary - 16% •

Q: 07
Do you believe that education and training is as prevalent for unbiased technology as for other types of technology?

The answers went like this:

Yes - 38% •
No - 54% •
Not necessary - 8% •

Q: 08
Have you seen or been aware of improper use of any technology where clients' skin has been damaged?

92% of skin professionals answered yes.

Q: 09
Do "more at risk" photo-types affect your confidence and choice of technology when it comes to your skin practice?

This was a relatively even split. 46% said that it did affect their confidence and choice of technology. 54% said that this didn't have an impact on their choices and confidence

Q: 10
Do you believe that there are readily available technologies for the skin professional that aligns with a multicultural/cross-cultural clientele demographic?

A completely even split on this one. 50/50.

WHAT THE RESULTS TELL US

These survey results are encouraging in some areas, and not-so encouraging in others. It's clear that there are some communities, professionals and clients that are simply not served by what's out there. This is extremely disappointing for everyone.

It does nothing for the industry and nothing for the clients at the end of it. 92% of skin professionals have had a client rock up with skin that's been damaged by the wrong technology. That is absolutely unacceptable and needs to change.

So how do we solve this problem? I believe that education is the answer for a lot of the issues and knowledge that's missing from the conversation. This needs to be embedded in training and education right from the beginning, so that cultural awareness and skin health equity is there from the start. It shouldn't be an afterthought or something to read up on later.

KEY TAKEAWAYS

- A better understanding of the conditions that affect darker skin, how to recognise them and how to treat them is needed.

- Positive progress is being made within the industry, which is exciting, necessary and long overdue.
- Darker skin isn't a contraindication and isn't 'difficult to treat'.

THE LASER DRAMA

*I*n this chapter, you'll learn about:

- The history of laser treatments in the industry.
- What to be aware of when it comes to lasers and melanin.
- The evolution of the laser industry.
- Laser options and alternatives for darker skin.
- The future of laser treatments.

WHAT'S ALL THE DRAMA?

If you regularly recommend laser treatments to your clients, then you *should* be well aware of how laser works and its suitability for different photo-types.

Maybe I'm preaching to the choir here. I kind of hope that I am. You might be thinking "yep, I get it...so what's the drama?"

Well, the drama comes with those professionals who *don't* get it. Who recommend the wrong type of laser treatments to their clients with dark skin, causing discomfort, damage and worry. Maybe drama is the wrong word. In this case, it's less dramatic and more *traumatic* for the client.

On the opposite side of the drama/trauma are the skin-care professionals who just flat-out suggest that laser isn't a suitable treatment for black skin. They turn away clients, provide no other options or advice and send them on their way.

In the middle of the drama are clients with darker skin who are left feeling unsure, uninformed and with the overarching belief that no lasers work for black skin.

Now, I'm all for giving the right advice to clients, and avoiding treatments or situations that aren't going to be right or effective for them. But remember what we said about skin health equity?

As per the last chapter you just read: **black skin *isn't* a contraindication**. Every skin type and tone deserves the most effective treatments, and the treatments that are safe for their skin.

Let's take it back to basics and learn more about laser (and using it with melanin-rich skin) to really get to the bottom of how it works, how to use it and how to avoid making mistakes.

THE HISTORY OF LASER

Laser technology's roots go all the way back to the 1900s, where scientists discovered the connection between energy and frequency of radiation. I'll run through how lasers work on the skin in a little more detail later on in this chapter.

I'll skip through the next 60 years of development of photon technology, polarization and quantum particles to get to the point where lasers are being used in skincare. That's really what we're here to talk about.

In 1960, US physicist Theodore Maiman developed a ruby rod laser to use in a clinical setting. This development led US surgeon Leon Goldman to pioneer in using lasers in dermatology. He was the first person to report the effects of the laser on destroying pigmented elements like dark hair.

Over the next 10 years or so there was a rush of development in the field. Lasers were used for things like tattoo removal, removal of skin lesions, wound healing and photodynamic therapy.

A big jump in laser technology came in the 90s. Robotic scanning technology was developed which meant that lasers could now be used in a more precise way across the skin. This meant no more going over the same area more than once, which could damage the skin.

These developments also meant that anti-aging and rejuvenating laser treatments became more possible.

In short, lasers have been used in skincare for around 40-50 years. There hasn't been any new technology in around 30-40 years. When you hear about "new lasers" on the market, it's really just the old technology with an upgrade. Interesting, right?

Lasers use heat and light on the same wavelength to achieve the desired result on the skin. They use crystal rods to determine the wavelength of the laser - this is important as in general, longer wavelength treatments are more suitable for darker skin. Short wavelengths tend to be more intense and can be more damaging on dark skin (we'll talk about that a little later in the chapter).

There are 10 different laser types operating under a number of different brand names. Although the underlying technology is the same, there's differences to how the machines work in a practical sense.

As a professional, you might have preferences on how certain laser brands work. That might be as simple as the weight and feel of it to use, or it might be down to the training and support that's given to you from the brand.

Now, lasers are used for a whole host of skin, aesthetic and beauty treatments across a variety of concerns. The technology is improving and developing but there are still some gaps. It's predominantly been a treatment that's been used for lighter skin, meaning that it's excluded a whole host of people looking to rejuvenate their skin and treat certain skin concerns.

For the longest time, for example, laser hair removal simply wasn't available to those with darker skin due to the way the technology worked to identify and remove hairs. It was offered on the basis that it worked best for "pale skin and dark hair". This is no longer the case and there are laser hair removal options that are suitable for dark skin, but until relatively recently it simply wasn't an option.

WHAT IS LASER USED FOR?

In terms of esthetics, laser treatments can be used for a whole range of different reasons. Here are some of the most popular:

- Laser hair removal.
- Fading hyperpigmentation.
- Reducing visible red blood vessels (also known as thread veins).
- Resurface the skin to improve the appearance of scarring or fine lines.
- Anti-aging.
- Skin conditions like rosacea.
- Improve skin texture.
- Reducing the appearance of large pores.
- Removing skin tags, lesions and unwanted growths from the skin.
- Promoting skin healing and health.
- Improving collagen production.

Laser treatments are also used for other non-skincare treatments such as tattoo removal, laser eye surgery and even teeth whitening. They're also used in surgery and in medical treatments too.

When used correctly and appropriately, laser treatments can make a huge difference to the appearance and condition of the skin, particularly as a targeted treatment.

Correctly and *appropriately* are the key points here. Using the wrong type of laser on some photo-types of skin is a recipe for disaster.

There's often a lot of confusion around laser treatments, what they do and how much down-time a client needs after a treatment.

I think that's because there are so many treatments out there that are badged as "laser" that work in completely different ways, and have different results. That's why one client may have loved their treatment, whereas another client at another venue hated theirs. They both had "laser" treatments but for completely different reasons, and with different types of laser.

Even treatments that aren't laser-based - like LED, UV, infra-red, IPL and microdermabrasion - sometimes get confused with laser treatments as the treatment experience can feel similar and targets similar concerns.

This leads to a situation where people recommend their "laser" treatment to others when…no lasers were actually used on their skin in the first place.

Phew! It's no wonder clients get confused about what they want sometimes. There are a ton of treatments out there and misinformation is everywhere unfortunately. Don't even get me started on clients who are recommended to try treatments that don't work and will do nothing for their skin.

Back to the truth about lasers. We'll run through the different types of lasers below, so that you can get to grips with how they work and what they do - as well as who they work for.

TYPES OF LASER

Broadly speaking, there are two different types of laser that are commonly used in skincare:

- Ablative laser treatments
- Non-ablative laser treatments

Both types of lasers work in slightly different ways, give different results and offer different healing processes. There are also differences in their suitability for some skin photo-types.

Ablative Laser Treatments

Ablative laser treatments remove the top layer of the skin with an intense laser light. They heat the underlying skin to stimulate the growth of new collagen fibers. You might also hear them referred to as CO_2 lasers or wounding lasers (eek).

They're most commonly used for wrinkles, deep scarring and skin rejuvenation. As the skin heals and regrows, the client will usually see smoother and tighter skin revealed. The results usually last 1-5 years.

This type of treatment is usually best for mild to moderate wrinkles and is best for clients who show signs of significant facial aging, have deep or pitted scars, want fast results and can take the time out to recover. Because...well, there is significant down time with this.

Because they remove the top layer of the skin, the down time is weeks rather than days. It can be up to two weeks of skin that's red, raw and a little oozy. It's important to ensure that your client is well aware of this fact before they head down that road.

Some of the brands of ablative laser treatments include CO_2 and the Erbium:YAG laser. There are lots of others on the market too, so do your research if you're planning a purchase.

In general, clients with darker skin tones should avoid ablative laser treatments as there's a risk with permanent hyperpigmentation that comes with it. More on that to come, but I believe that's where laser treatments get their bad rep for black skin from.

Non-Ablative Laser Treatments

Non-ablative lasers don't break the surface of your skin. They're usually gentler than ablative treatments and require less downtime.

These types of laser treatments are also better for improving skin texture and tone. They may also work for mild hyperpigmentation, wrinkles, sun-damaged skin or minor dark spots.

They're often used for clients that have mild to moderate signs of aging, want to skip a long recovery time and are happy to undergo multiple treatments. It also helps the skin to generate collagen.

The recovery time for non-ablative treatments is shorter (usually more like 4-5 days in total) as they're less damaging on all skin types and tones. The results are usually long-lasting too, again 3-5 years.

CoolTouch, Fraxel Restore and N-Lite are all types of non-ablative lasers, but there are other brands out there too.

I have previously seen excellent results for laser treatments on dark skin with the Nd:Yag laser system. It targets the blood supply that's attached to the hair follicle, rather than the difference in pigment to the skin. It penetrates more deeply into the skin to get to - quite literally - the root of the problem, rather than the surface. It does heat the follicle slightly, but it's absorption into melanin is poor, unlike other laser types. It doesn't affect the natural melanin in the skin and is therefore more suitable for darker skin, when the correct wavelength is used. As with all treatments, safety and testing precautions should always be taken with each client.

Other Types of Laser

There are some other types of lasers that are used commercially too. The underlying technology works in the same way but with some key differences.

Fractional laser is a type of laser treatment that directs a laser beam that's split into thousands of microscopic treatment zones. It leaves tiny, microscopic spaces between the light that touches the skin, meaning that less skin is exposed to the laser, areas aren't "re-lasered" during a treatment but you still get the rejuvenating benefits where the light touches. They're so close together that it isn't like "you missed a spot", it just means less skin is affected by the laser. It can be more gentle and just as effective.

Picosecond laser uses very short pulses of light and is usually used to remove tattoos, though they can also be used to remodel the skin, treating signs of aging, sun damage and acne scarring.

Q-Switch laser creates a light beam that pulses (pretty much invisibly), which means that the light isn't continuously on your skin. Again, it's common for tattoo removal but can also be used to remove lesions, deal with pigmentation issues and for skin rejuvenation.

There are also at-home "laser" treatments available, but these are unlikely to give the same results as more effective, professional treatments. These definitely do need to be handled with caution, however, especially when it comes to darker skin. There are far too many horror stories of use-at-home lasers on darker skin, which is why I strongly recommend against it.

SKIN THEOLOGIAN'S TIP

Confusingly, some brands also offer ablative and non-ablative laser treatments under their brand. This kind of adds to the confusion if someone mentions that they "had a Fraxel treatment" (Fraxel is a brand of laser treatment), they could mean Fraxel DUAL, Fraxel Restore or Fraxel Re:Pair.

They all sound similar, right? So What's the difference?

Fraxel Restore and Fraxel DUAL are **non-ablative** laser treatments commonly used to resurface the skin. As non-ablative treatments, they're more suitable for a range of skin tones. However, Fraxel Re:Pair is a more aggressive, **ablative** laser treatment that isn't likely to be suitable for dark skin.

Again: it's no wonder people get confused.

I'm not singling out Fraxel in particular here, lots of laser brands offer both types. I just wanted to educate you and make sure you understand just how important it is to be clear on what treatments you're offering and what their suitability is. You heard that a certain brand was good for dark skin? Well, make sure you're clear on which treatment is the right one.

THE DOWNSIDES OF LASER (FOR ALL CLIENTS)

I'm here to bring you a balanced, experienced viewpoint on what skincare's all about. Whilst laser can be an effective treatment, there are some downsides too (like pretty much everything), and it's important that you understand these as a professional:

- The downtime needed for some types of treatment.

- You will need specialist training, and probably specialist insurance, equipment and premises.
- It can be expensive (both as a professional investing in training and equipment, and as a client).
- Clients usually need multiple treatments to see results with some types of laser (not necessarily a downside).
- Some types of laser aren't suitable for all different photo-types of skin - this may mean investing in more than one type of equipment.
- There can be side effects like redness, infection, scarring or skin color changes.
- There's usually aftercare that needs to be followed. No type of laser is a one-and-done treatment that will offset a poor routine or lack of ongoing care.
- There are limitations to what can be achieved - we've all had clients who expect that one skincare treatment will change their life. Sometimes that's the case, sometimes they may need to readjust their expectations to discover what's actually realistic.

SKIN THEOLOGIAN'S TIP

Let's jump back a little and think about where we've talked about cultural intelligence. It's linked to honesty, awareness and your role as a professional.

Something else that's important - and not necessarily linked to cultural intelligence *directly*, but absolutely in the same ballpark is this:

You're the expert.

Your clients are coming to you for your knowledge, expertise and skills. They're paying you for that knowledge and the service.

Part of this honesty also comes with being honest about the anticipated results of a treatment. I mentioned above about laser limitations and being realistic with clients.

We've all had clients who are expecting the results of a facelift in a bottle (if you haven't, lucky you!), which isn't realistic.

Sometimes the misconceptions come as a result of media hype, another skin pro who's not been totally honest or a mix up in before and after images. I.e. they're referring to the results of a surgical procedure, but they're here for a skin-care routine.

Be honest with your clients. Don't be afraid to have those open and honest conversations. Don't undersell your services, but make sure they're not left feeling disappointed or underwhelmed about their results.

Make sure they understand the impacts of life-style and proper aftercare too, or the fact they may need multiple treatments.

Of course, there are extremely effective treatments available, and for some clients these are literally life changing. For others, they'll leave the treatment disappointed. This could affect your professional reputation.

LASER VS DARK SKIN

When it comes to laser and darker skin, not all treatments have been created equally. It's extremely important to understand what these differences are and how to work with your client's skin so that you're able to offer far more skin health equity than some types of treatment do (looking at you, ablative laser treatments).

Unfortunately people seem to fall into two camps when it comes to a lack of awareness about laser:

1. "Black skin can't have laser treatments. Sorry and goodbye."
2. "I'm going to do this treatment on black skin anyway and then be incredibly surprised to see that it's actually caused long-term, negative effects."

Both of these attitudes are rooted in extreme ignorance of how to work with darker skin tones. Neither of these attitudes express an *ounce* of skin health equity, but number 2 would probably tell you that they were being inclusive and treating everyone the same.

We know the drill now: that's *not* what skin health equity is about at all. Everyone is different, and that needs to be taken into account so that people can have the best skin of their lives. Remember, celebrating differences goes hand in hand with celebrating similarities.

Let's have an open conversation about lasers and dark skin.

The Truth About Lasers and Melanin-Rich Skin

Not all laser and light therapies are safe for every skin tone, especially when it comes to darker skin. In general, skin that's above type IV on the Fitzpatrick scale (more on that to come in the next chapter - I've got some thoughts about *that* particular measurement) need to be careful when it comes to laser.

It's essential that - as a professional - you understand this, understand how lasers work and know what to tell your client. Inexperienced practitioners cause damage to dark skin. There, I said it. It's true.

There are some lasers that are safe for dark skin. Mainly long wavelength lasers, rather than the short wavelength ablative laser treatments.

The short explanation is that most esthetic lasers target water, red hemoglobin or brown melanin in the skin. This is how the laser identified what to target and to remove pigment.

Darker skin contains more melanin than lighter skin tones, which means that some types of laser aren't as effective or that it targets the skin differently, causing damage. It's really another example of dark skin being an afterthought during the development of laser esthetic treatments, just like in other parts of the industry.

When used incorrectly, laser can have some terrible effects on dark skin, including:

- Pain.
- Burns.
- Scars.
- Hypopigmentation.
- Hyperpigmentation.
- Long-term skin damage.

It's serious stuff, and I don't take this conversation lightly at all. Laser has a bad rep in the black community for this exact reason. Incorrect treatments, poor training and a lack of education all lead to this situation. It's yet another example of skin inequity. *Le sigh.*

The survey that I carried out with skin care professionals showed that there's a lack of adequate training when it comes to dealing with the outcomes of skin that's been damaged by photo or thermal treatments (like laser). Almost 70% of skin professionals said that they hadn't received adequate training to support them to understand the recovery time for this type of damage. This becomes a cycle of damage that leaves the customer feeling worried and underwhelmed.

92% of skin professionals I surveyed had seen damaged skin as a result of use of improper technology. When you put those two statistics together it makes something of a worrying picture.

Which Types Of Laser Are Safe For Dark Skin?

It's not all bad news, however. There are a whole host of laser treatments that are safer for dark skin. I still say handle with care and I absolutely recommend doing your own research - technology and guidance changes all of the time. This isn't a cut-and-dried list, it's a guide for you to head off and do your more in-depth research on the types of laser out there, and who they're best suited to.

I'm not affiliated with any of these laser brands in any way as my approach is always to offer education that's unbiased to any line or brand of technology, and as I said, I urge you to do your own research in what laser treatments to pick up, but here's a guide to lasers which are generally considered better for dark skin:

- Non ablative laser treatments (like Clear + Brilliant Fraxel DUAL and Lutronic Ultra).
- Picosecond lasers (like Enlighten, Pico Genesis, PicoSure and PicoWay).
- YAG lasers go deeper into the skin and bypass pigmentation so are safer for darker skin. An example is the Nd:YAG that I referenced earlier.
- Diode laser treatments usually need to be

delivered more slowly, using the right device to avoid damage on dark skin, and has an instant cooling function to reduce damage. An example is LightSheer Diode Laser.

You want to avoid traditional, resurfacing treatments that use ablative lasers - such as some types of Fraxel and CO2 devices. These are more likely to damage dark skin, leaving it with permanent hyperpigmentation or damage.

Shoutout to Intense Pulsed Light (IPL) and Broadband Light (BBL) treatments too. These are often commonly linked in conversation with laser, but neither are truly safe for dark skin. It's likely that clients with darker skin will see complications from these treatments. You need to be using specific technology that works best for darker skin tones.

SKIN THEOLOGIAN'S TIP

Wondering how to have a CQ conversation with a potential client about laser? Let's set the scene:

A potential client comes in to discuss laser. This potential client is black. The laser treatments that you offer aren't the most suitable for dark skin.

What do you do next? And how do you have a conversation with the client that lets them know what you can offer isn't right for them, without it feeling like a brush off?

Let's talk about what you shouldn't do next, first.

1. Don't just wave them away and say "oh we can't deal with *your* skin here."

2. Don't carry out the treatment regardless.

The best way to handle this situation is to be open and honest about the facts. The treatment you offer is likely to damage their skin. You don't want that and neither do they.

Take it as an opportunity to educate them about the treatments that *are* suitable for their skin - that could be alternatives that you offer (make sure you outline results, process, safety and how effective each treatment is) or it could involve referring them elsewhere. The conversation should be culturally intelligent, open and kind. It should be framed as coming from a place of care and expertise, not exclusion and even personal opinion.

Sometimes, what starts out as a mistake or an opinion becomes thought of as being factual.

This is how some of the biggest misnomers in skincare are still touted as the truth today. If you utilize your professional expertise rather than personal opinion, it's a start towards raising standards in the industry.

Make sure you *know* the score for the lasers you offer in advance. There's nothing that will diminish a client's confidence in you than you having to Google an answer, ring a supplier or hurriedly try to flip through a manual. This is not the impression you want to give as an expert that they're paying for to work on their skin.

In my opinion, having more than one technology on hand (or a type of laser that's suitable for a wider range of skin tones) is the best solution.

I realize there's a little nuance here.

Earlier I said "don't turn people away" and now I'm saying to send people elsewhere? That's part of CQ. Tailoring, adapting and being ready to perceive the bigger picture.

Inclusion is not about damaging skin for the sake of feeling too awkward to say otherwise.

It's actually more inclusive to educate and tailor your approach accordingly. It's never a static process, and is always an evolution.

ALTERNATIVES TO LASER

If you don't offer laser treatments, don't intend to and don't want to, but still want to have rejuvenating and resurfacing treatments available for your dark-skinned clients, then there are options. These can be a good way to offer skin health equity in-salon, provided that you're educated, experienced and understand what you're recommending.

These include:

- Light skin peels.
- Light microdermabrasion.
- Retinoids (be careful with these).
- Consistent skincare routine.
- Lifestyle changes.

The treatment portion of that list needs to be handled with care when it comes to dark skin, to avoid damage like inflammation and hyperpigmentation. It's important - actually, it's essential - to do a full consultation, and to take it slow.

THE FUTURE OF LASER

As I mentioned at the beginning of this chapter, much of the technology behind laser treatments hasn't changed a great deal since the 1960s. Whilst there's been progress, adaptations and improvements, it's mainly been based on that existing technology that was adapted by Theodore Maiman.

There are some interesting and exciting conversations going on in the laser world right now, to see how they can be used even further in skincare.

There's talk of laser being used to allow for tailored treatments and the introduction of skincare delivery using laser - such as *Hydroquinone*, antioxidants, platelet-rich plasma and post-procedural skincare regimens being delivered directly into the skin via laser. Topical treatments post-laser treatment are already used to allow them to penetrate the epidermis, this would just take it a little further.

Another opportunity for laser treatments in skin care is artificial intelligence (AI). Already used across the beauty industry, AI could be used to help guide laser treatments, show potential results, analyze skin, mix custom products, drive automation and to improve treatment safety.

One concern I have with this type of development is skin health equity. I've already mentioned issues with AI development and it's lack of diversity in development teams and the way the programs learn. For skincare, it would be even more essential that the machine's algorithms are programmed based on every available skin tone and shade. People with darker skin shouldn't be an afterthought in the beauty industry, regardless of whoever is creating the software.

And finally, highest on my wishlist is a laser treatment that's as effective and as suitable for every single skin tone out there.

USING LASER AS A SKIN PRO

If you want to add laser treatments to your roster, there are some things that you definitely need to be aware of.

Some of these tips are the same, whatever treatment type we're talking about as professionals, but they completely bear repeating when it comes to laser:

- Education is key. Get the best education you can on using lasers on your clients of all skin types and photo-types. Take the time to invest in working with the most knowledgeable and experienced trainers.

- Understand what types of lasers can be used on what types of skin. Offer alternative options if your laser isn't the right choice for their skin. Whether this is another trusted professional who can help them, or a different type of treatment. Let's leave "we can't treat your skin" in the dust.
- Invest in the right equipment. Laser equipment is expensive. I get that. But the right equipment means that you can start to generate a return on your investment, achieve results for your clients and work safely on their skin.
- If you offer laser treatment that's safe for darker skin, let people know. Make sure it's on your website, price lists and social media.Also, include the fact that you/your team are adequately trained to work safely on all photo-types and committed to constant learning. Save those prospective clients time and make your job far easier when it comes to getting new business.
- Update your knowledge. It's *too* easy to pass a training course and then never update your skills or knowledge of a treatment area. I shouldn't have to explain why this isn't the right idea when you're working with a client's skin.
- Practice and be confident. "Practice makes

perfect" might be an oldie, but it makes a good point. I like to say "practice makes permanent". What you practice will become your norm. In the interests of skin health equity, try and practice (safely) on different skin tones/photo-types where possible.

- Ensure that your training allows you to be fully licensed to carry out the treatment. Depending on where you are in the world, laws and regulations are different. Make sure you're up to date. In Canada, for instance, there is a lack of standardization across the provinces. This is being worked on, as it has been a hindrance to standards of excellence for far too long.

- Make sure your professional insurance covers laser treatments. It's always a good idea to periodically check that you're covered for everything you need to be and that you're practicing within the terms of your insurance. You don't want to find out that you're not when you try to use it.

- Patch test. Again, some insurance will require it. Even if they don't, your client's safety and treatment outcome are important.

- Carry out a full consultation with your client. In-person is best, so that you can really examine their skin, but this isn't always possible at the moment so make sure you're thorough in your questioning.

- Be prepared for the question "do you have experience in treating people with my skin color?" As mentioned earlier, unfortunately many clients out there believe that you have to look like them in order to be able to treat them. That's simply not the case.

- Keep a record of treatments. Again, this is usually a good idea for consistency and insurance purposes. It can also help you to spot patterns and plan treatments effectively. Plus, it's a more professional experience for your client.

- Advise on aftercare. Make sure they understand the importance.

- Listen to your client. If they're experiencing pain or discomfort, or telling you that something doesn't feel right, listen to them. Everyone has different tolerances, experiences and pain thresholds. You're relying on them to tell you how they feel, so you should listen.

As you can see, the topic of lasers and dark skin is a fairly detailed one. There's a lot of misinformation, misunderstandings and mistakes at every stage. I wasn't kidding when I called this chapter "The Laser Drama" as it truly does feel like that at times.

KEY TAKEAWAYS

- Lasers are not always the way forward for darker skin tones and weren't originally created with dark skin in mind.
- For lasers ideally suited for darker skin, look for non-ablative, longer wavelength laser options.
- There are alternatives to laser treatments that give similar rejuvenating effects without the damage.
- Keep your education up to date when it comes to lasers.

*__Note From Char__: "JUST CHECKING IN WITH YOU. Do you have questions or comments so far? Let me know on IG: @theskintheologian"

4

HEY FITZ! A CRITICAL LOOK AT THE FITZPATRICK SCALE

*I*n this chapter, you'll learn about:

- What the Fitzpatrick Scale is and how it works.
- The problem(s) with the Fitzpatrick Scale.
- What other options are there?
- How to have a culturally intelligent conversation around skin tones.

WHAT IS THE FITZPATRICK SCALE?

For the uninitiated (and according to the survey results we discussed earlier in the book that could be more than 75% of you who haven't been trained on skin photo types or don't feel that you need to), here's an introduction to the Fitzpatrick Scale.

The Fitzpatrick Scale is a way of classifying skin photo-types into categories, mainly in relation to their risk of sunburn and skin cancer. As we mentioned earlier in the book, skin with more melanin is less prone to sunburn (but not immune - keep recommending and wearing SPF, whatever your Fitpatrick category).

It was developed by Thomas B. Fitzpatrick, MD, PhD, in 1975 to assess the propensity of the skin to burn during phototherapy to assist him in choosing the correct dose of UVA energy in treatment for skin diseases.

It's often used by dermatologists, the medical community and some skincare specialists. It isn't usually used in makeup, but is sometimes used to assess clinical benefits and efficacy of cosmetic procedures.

It's even been used by the US's Homeland Security department, until they were advised to stop using it as it's too blunt an instrument that doesn't work with the diverse population in the US. Yet it is still being used elsewhere, and in particular the skin care industry, where it's been used for almost fifty years.

Here's a summary of the the Fitzpatrick Scale categories as they currently stand:

Type	Features of unexposed skin	Tanning and burning
1	very pale white skin, often with green or blue eyes and fair or red hair	burns without tanning
2	white skin, often with blue eyes	burns and does not tan easily
3	fair skin with brown eyes and brown hair	burns first then tans
4	light brown skin, dark eyes, and dark hair	burns a little and tans easily

5	brown skin, dark eyes, and dark hair	easily tans to a darker color and rarely burns
6	dark brown or black skin, dark eyes, and dark hair	never burns but tans darker

In the past there have been more comprehensive scales that have existed (check out Von Luschan's Chromatic Scale, this used glass slides to "measure" skin color which I don't really know how I feel about) but these weren't always reliable so ended up being abandoned.

THE PROBLEM(S) WITH THE FITZPATRICK SCALE

So, what's my problem with Fitz? I said I was all for skin health equity, I want all skin tones to receive the right care for their skin and I want professionals to use their expertise and knowledge to treat darker skin correctly.

Surely there needs to be something that differentiates the different tones and shades from one another? How else are you meant to work out where someone's shade fits in?

Well, grab a seat, settle down and we'll talk through some of the limitations, problems and issues with the Fitzpatrick Scale. I'm going to be honest with you, to me the Fitzpatrick scale just isn't really fitting when it comes to skin of color. Here's my thoughts on the topic:

It's extremely general

Obviously there will always be exceptions to every category, rule or grouping of people but - where do you fit in if you have brown skin, green eyes and natural red hair? What if you have lighter skin but don't burn easily? A personal, expert assessment of the skin is always better than slotting someone into a category, but I do understand that it's often being used as a starting point.

It's very subjective

Every decision we make and every thought we have is related to our own experiences. It's the same with the Fitzpatrick Scale. What's light-skinned to me, might be dark to someone else and vice versa. It relies on interpretation, and that interpretation is going to come with some sort of bias. This means that it's applied inconsistently across the medical progression.

It was designed for UV sensitivity

As I mentioned, when the Fitzpatrick Scale was first created it was used as a classification around UV sensitivity for medical treatment. It wasn't designed as a "catch-all" skin color scale. This has now become a means of describing skin color and ethnicity in health and medical conversations that are unrelated to sunburn, skin cancer and tanning. This is likely to be just because there was nothing else.

Types 5 and 6 weren't initially included

When the scale was created in 1975, it only included photo types 1-4. There was no place on the scale where dark skin was included. It might not surprise you to learn that Thomas B. Fitzpatrick is probably a 1 or 2 skin photo type on his scale. Categories 5 and 6 were added later. This is another example of widely-used medical tools that have been founded upon a biased approach without cultural inclusivity at its core.

Race, ethnicity and pigmentation aren't all the same

Many physicians who use the Fitzpatrick scale use it as a correlation with race. But people self-report differently. Japanese women often self-identify as type 2, but Asian skin is often classified as different to fair skin. So where does that fit in?

It doesn't take into account skin changes

Most skin types change color throughout the seasons. More sun exposure means darker skin, whereas in winter (when it feels like the sun disappears) skin gets lighter. FYI - that winter color is known as constitutive skin and describes skin that's free from external factors like sunlight. Conversely, skin conditions like hyper-pigmentation, melasma or rosacea change the skin's appearance and shade - does that mean that person belongs in a different Fitzpatrick category?

Skin color is different across the body

Having different shades across your body is completely normal, and something that everyone has. Some people's face, neck and chest are three completely different shades. These differences can be significant. So if you're carrying out a body treatment that needs to take into account skin shade, and that's different on certain parts of the body, which point on the scale should you use? I think you may be starting to get my point...

It hinders CQ conversations

The ability to just quietly categorize someone as a certain skin photo-type without needing to have that "awkward" conversation (I promise it doesn't have to be awkward and I'll discuss that later on in this chapter) about skin color and skin concerns is actually doing your clients a disservice. It probably means that their needs aren't really being met, which to me is *way* more awkward than an open and honest CQ conversation.

It depersonalizes the client

"You're a 6", "you're a 2", "hmm, you might be a 5 I guess?". Have you ever experienced a situation where being treated like a number rather than a person has been a positive thing? I thought not! Everyone is their own person with thoughts, opinions and experiences - they should be treated that way.

Linking UV sensitivity to skin concerns doesn't always work

Sometimes, systems designed with the best of intentions don't work as intended. By categorizing skin color in a way that's aligned with UV sensitivity, it can mask real skin conditions. It's a fact that people with darker skin tones who have skin cancer (the most common type that black people experience is squamous cell carcinoma whereas basal cell carcinoma is more popular in Asian and Hispanic people) are more likely to have their cancer diagnosis at a later stage, lessening survival rates, because of the myth that "people with dark skin don't get cancer".

SKIN THEOLOGIAN'S TIP

Let's pause and talk about skin cancer for a second. As I mentioned, skin cancer is often missed or diagnosed at a much later stage in people of color because of the perception that skin cancer shouldn't be a concern as the risk is so low.

Darker skin - in fact any skin - can experience skin cancer. Usually caused by sun exposure without protection, it's not exclusive to those with lighter skin. This is a misconception that exists both within communities of color and outside of them. And it's causing harm.

I recently came across an astounding piece on the presence of Melanoma cases among those of darker skin.

A variant of Melanoma can be quite commonly found in those of darker skin tones. It can be experienced on parts of the skin that are exposed to the sun, but aren't even thought about for sun protection, such as the feet and the hands.

Acral Lentiginous Melanoma of the foot is a relatively rare but often very aggressive variant of Melanoma. More commonly identified in patients with darker skin, diagnosis of the lesions is often delayed because the area is not routinely examined by patients or primary care physicians".

It is time for this misconception to be dispelled that by the shade or tone of one's skin, one can be exempt from fatal diseases. The great news is, if caught early, it can be 100% reversible!

This is where education is fundamental! If we can help to spread the word on the prevalence of Melanoma, the risks to all skin (including dark skin), and the value of regular checks from skin professionals, we could literally save someone's life.

I told you I had some thoughts on this topic! I think any method of measuring or categorizing skin color will always have some sort of limitation to it. Often, the system is only as good as the person using it. Research has shown that use of the Fitzpatrick scale alongside an actual medical examination of the skin leads to a more accurate treatment in dermatology.

Skin comes in so many different shades (even on the same person) that fitting them into one of six categories is *never* going to be straightforward. When makeup brands are releasing foundation ranges with 50+ different shades, and there are *still* some people who are in between, six is just not going to cut it.

Whilst I'm on the topic of makeup, skin tones and skin health equity, let's just talk marketing for a second. When you see a product advertised - a product to tackle hyperpigmentation for example - and it says "90% of people said their brown spots faded within weeks", there's no way of knowing how diverse and representative that cross-section was. It might mean it was tested on Fitzpatrick types 1-4 only, so no-one has any idea of what happens on 5-6. Of course it could be the other way around, but let's be honest: there are still too many additional factors to take into account here.

Moving back to assessing skin phototypes, In the next section, we'll talk about some alternatives to the Fitz-patrick scale when it comes to assessing skin color and tailoring skin care treatments appropriately.

SKIN THEOLOGIAN'S TIP

This is probably more of a "tip-off" than a tip but I wanted to talk about where I think the move from "UV treatment categorization" through to "all-purpose skin color grading system" came from.

I actually think the shift might have been when lasers started to become popularized (there goes that drama again! What is it with laser?!) and the categories were hijacked by the laser industry in conversations around light therapy suitability and pigment. I can't prove this, but the theory fits. What's funny is that most lasers don't even use UV light in any capacity, so it uses a reference point the Fitzpatrick scale) that refers to a completely different system. Does that make much sense?

The fact that 77% of survey respondents said that they were trained on Fitzpatrick in relation to thermal and light-emitting treatments does seem to back this theory up somewhat.

ALTERNATIVES TO THE FITZPATRICK SCALE

If not the Fitzpatrick scale, then what? How do we ensure that darker skin receives appropriate treatment for their particular shade and skin concerns, without categorizing it so broadly?

One of the most prominent options right now is scanning technology that uses AI to identify an exact shade match. This has been used across the makeup and beauty sector by a number of different brands, mostly to match makeup and products for purchase.

There are real opportunities for skin professionals to use this in their practice to identify skin concerns, pigmentation issues and accurately photo type skin if that's needed. Some of the AI systems that are being used in dermatology can achieve accuracy that is on par with US board-certified dermatologists, as shown in studies.

Even tech giant Google are currently developing an inclusive, light-based alternative to the Fitzpatrick Scale. They're working in collaboration with scientific and medical experts, along with groups working with communities of color, to develop tools built with skin health equity in mind.

This came about after Google launched a new AI dermatology tool, using the Fitzpatrick Scale. They quickly realized the scale was inadequate and somewhat outdated. As a result they're now working on new ways to recognize and classify skin phototypes. They're committing themselves to diversify their image datasets and to create a guidebook to capture skin tones to improve how the algorithms work.

Interesting, right? When I said that I didn't think the Fitzpatrick Scale was up to scratch, I knew I was in good company. It isn't, and there needs to be a better way.

HOW TO HAVE A CQ CONVERSATION AROUND SKIN TONES

I've highlighted that it's important to treat darker skin tones and skin concerns appropriately throughout the book. This means that you'll need to address skin tones and concerns with your clients. However, I've also said not to just lean on the six category Fitzpatrick Scale as a way to assign treatments to a client. It's too broad and not inclusive enough. Dark skin comes in hundreds of different shades - as does lighter skin - so to lump every melanin-rich skin tone into "5" or "6" seems disingenuous. It's doing your clients a disservice.

Both of these points can be correct, and I believe that they are. **By no longer using the Fitzpatrick Scale as a crutch in the conversation, you can actually have a much more useful, open conversation with your client that embodies CQ.**

Where to start when it comes to what words to use when discussing skin tone with your clients...

Before we jump right in, I think it's important to give a bit of context.

Language is a beautiful instrument of communication. Although it is an instrument, it is *not* the only instrument. There is touch, body language, facial expressions and so on.

We've all heard that the words hold power. I have always believed this myself to be true, and I still believe this.

A few years ago I discovered something equally important as the words that I choose to use in both my professional and personal life.

The intentions behind or "spirit" of the words that are used.

Before you dismiss this as too intangible, consider the following. Have you ever done a kind gesture for someone and they received it with heartfelt gratitude and gave you a tearful, heartfelt "thank you"? You can feel the spirit behind that "thank you", can't you?

And if you did the same kind gesture for someone else, who did not appreciate it, but felt the need to give you an obligatory "thank you", you can feel that too! Both people used the exact same words. But both were delivered in two very different ways that came across loud and clear (even when the intent was silent). The vehicle of gratitude and the other, the vehicle of ingratitude.

Words do hold power. They are vehicles for something much, much deeper; *Intention*!

And so, although you may want to choose the correct words, when discussing skin concerns with culturally diverse clients, it doesn't just stop with what you say. It's also how you say it.

Are your mindset and intentions coming from a place of (CQ) or are they coming from a place of fear and apprehension? Clients in fact, *people*, can feel that. Believe me.

Having said that, there are a wide range of words that are appropriate in different parts of the globe. Trying to distinguish a set amount of fool-proof words is not realistic. My standard guideline is to listen (*really listen*) to your clients' way of communicating.

If you're really not sure how to have that conversation, you can level up your knowledge by doing some additional research and reading. Referring to melanin-rich skin is usually helpful - all skin contains melanin, just darker skin contains a denser quality.

My tips for this conversation are similar to those that I outlined in Chapter 2. Approach these conversations with CQ, professionalism and kindness. I'd like to also add a little point here about professional language and how it comes across to the client.

Demonstrating technical expertise and knowledge is important, and it's important to speak to your clients in a professional manner. However, you should avoid jargon or information that may be meaningful to you, that a client won't understand.

For example, if you use the Fitzpatrick Scale when reviewing treatment options for your clients and you refer to them by their Fitzpatrick category, this isn't likely to mean anything to the client whatsoever. It may mean that they feel like they're just a number on a conveyor belt of treatments, or they might misunderstand it for some other unit of measurement. Talk in terms of their actual skin and their skin care needs.

If you don't use the Fitzpatrick Scale, but don't feel comfortable talking about different shades and skin tones, then this will likely come across in your treatment. A client will pick up on that discomfort, in the same way that they may have picked up on these types of invisible cues throughout their whole lives.

KEY TAKEAWAYS

- The Fitzpatrick Scale is seriously overdue for an update and isn't relevant in many situations.
- Technology will be the way forward when it comes to finding an alternative.
- CQ is essential in the conversation with the client.

5

REVIEW OF COMMON SKIN CONCERNS WITH DARKER SKIN

*I*n this chapter, you'll learn about:

- The types of skin conditions that are more prevalent in black skin.
- Why darker skin, professional treatments and advanced treatments go hand-in-hand.
- How to discuss skin conditions with CQ.

WHAT YOU NEED TO KNOW ABOUT SKIN CONDITIONS IN DARKER SKIN

As a skin professional, you'll be well-versed in a range of different skin conditions and how to treat them. When it comes to working with darker skin tones there are a few things you need to keep in mind:

- Some skin conditions will present differently on darker skin.
- Some treatments and skincare ingredients may not be effective or safe for darker skin.
- Many skincare resources don't address the differences, and you may find it difficult to even find reference images of some skin conditions on darker skin (I know I did).
- Just like all skin, not all darker skin is the same, so you need to use your professional expertise and skills.
- Ignore the skin myths you've heard about black skin and take the time to educate yourselves on these.
- There are some skin conditions that are more prevalent in darker skin.

There are a whole lot of myths and misconceptions with darker skin, which we've talked about, and it's important to remember that darker skin still comes in the same skin types and experiences the same skin conditions as lighter skin.

Darker skin will still show signs of aging, can get burned in the sun and can suffer from dehydration or congestion. Those things aren't different.

There are however some skin conditions that are more common in people with darker skin.

SKIN CONDITIONS THAT ARE MORE PREVALENT IN DARKER SKIN

As I mentioned above, there are some skin conditions that are more prevalent in darker skin. However, that *isn't* to say that they only affect dark skin so whoever your client is and whatever they look like, you need to find out about their skin. Some of these conditions were referenced in Volume 1 but are certainly worth attention with some expansion in this work as well.

A thorough consultation, asking the right questions, will help you to determine what you're working with (and therefore how to treat it or whether it needs to be referred elsewhere).

Here are some of the common skin conditions that you may find in clients with darker skin. Take the time to read up on these conditions - including imagery - to ensure that you're prepared and you know what to look for.

Acral Lentiginous Melanoma

This Melanoma cancer variant goes highly undetected in darker skin, usually until it's too late for treatment.

This links to the perception that darker skin contains natural SPF. It's also important to consider that someone's cultural identity may also have different heritage in their background, which can mean that there's less melanin in their skin. Familiarize yourself with what this variant looks like on darker skin, and if you have concerns ensure that your client refers themselves for medical investigation as soon as possible. You may save a life.

Dermatosis Papulosa Nigra

Dermatosis Papulosa Nigra presents as small, benign skin lesions and bumps on the skin. They're usually smooth, round and flat but can also look a little like a skin tag.

They're thought to be genetic and cause no harm, but many people dislike their appearance and may look to have them removed. Treatments include curettage, electrocautery, cryosurgery and laser Scarring, hyperpigmentation and keloids can all be a potential side-effect of removal, so they need to be handled with care and dealt with by someone who is experienced in using the right treatments for darker skin.

Around one third of the black population experiences Dermatosis Papulosa Nigra as they age, and it's considerably more common for those with darker skin to experience this.

Eczema

Eczema is believed to occur twice as frequently in children with darker skin (which is often when this condition starts). Often, eczema is misdiagnosed initially, so you may have a client present to you with "dry skin" who actually has undiagnosed eczema. It's important for you as a professional to understand what this condition looks like on darker skin.

Ideally, eczema needs a medical diagnosis and medical treatment, particularly if it's severe, painful or the skin is cracked. You should use your professional judgment to decide whether or not a client presenting with eczema has contraindications for their treatment. I.e. weeping, open or cracked patches.

If it's not diagnosed or treated, then it can cause issues with pigmentation or scarring, usually from itching or skin cracking.

Hidradenitis Suppurativa

Hidradentis Suppurativa (sometimes known as acne inversa) is an inflammatory skin disease that causes painful lumps and scarring, usually where skin rubs together like the armpit or groin. It's almost twice as common in the black community than other groups.

This is a medical condition that needs treatment. If a client presents to you with this condition, it's usually a contraindication to treatment if you're working on the area that's affected.

Hyperpigmentation

Hyperpigmentation is one of the biggest concerns when it comes to darker skin. It's dark patches or spots on the skin caused by inflammation, sun damage, scarring, insect bites, piercings, surgical incisions, acne or hormones that have resulted in an overproduction of melanin as the area heals.

Darker skin can show hyperpigmentation more visibly than other skin types. Be careful with treatment as some products and treatments (such as hydroquinone, which is often recommended as this can cause further pigmentation to the skin).

Hypertrophic scarring

A hypertrophic scar is a thick raised scar that's an abnormal response to wound healing. It's caused by excess collagen being produced during the healing process.

They more commonly occur in taut skin areas following skin trauma, burns or surgical incisions. Treatments include medication, freezing, injections, lasers and surgery. They do not usually extend beyond the original would.

Ichthyosis

This genetic skin condition is characterized by dry, thickened and scaly skin. It ranges in severity, symptoms and the underlying genetic cause. It can be itchy, dry and painful. This would generally be considered a contraindication to most skin care treatments due to damaging the skin.

Keloid scarring

Keloid scars are raised scarring and lumps on the skin that may have discoloration, redness or irritation. It's an overreaction to wound healing and scarring, caused by the production of too many fibroblasts in the skin. The scar keeps growing, even after the wound is healed and can end up being larger than the wound that caused it. This is what distinguishes it from a hypertrophic scar; the scar extends beyond the borders of the original wound. Hypertrophic scars do not.

Keloid scarring can appear on any type of skin, but is more common on darker skin. Some research believes it relates to too much collagen being produced during the healing process after a piercing, injury or surgical incision.

They can usually be removed by a medical professional, but can come back worse than before as a reaction. They aren't a treatment contraindication for non-invasive treatments, but you should make sure that you're careful with areas that have keloid scarring and make sure that your client is comfortable.

It's important to always ask about keloid scarring with your clients during their consultation, especially if you're doing any treatments that puncture or pierce the skin.

Keratosis Pilaris

This commonly goes hand in hand with eczema and ichthyosis, both of which are more common in darker skin. It gives the appearance of goosebumps (or 'chicken skin'), most commonly around thighs and the tops of your arms. It isn't painful or contagious, but can be annoying. It's caused by hair follicles producing too much keratin.

Exfoliation and hydration are two of the treatments to deal with this skin condition. Warm baths and avoiding tight clothing can also keep it at bay.

Lichenification

This is a harmless condition but is often the result of other skin conditions such as eczema or dermatitis. Lichenification can be caused by stress and consists of excessive itching or rubbing, resulting in an irritable rash.

It is treatable and the skin can return to normal once the inflammation is kept under control but it can be difficult to identify in black skin and is often confused with fungal infections. This is often a contraindication to treatment that needs medical attention to clear up.

Melasma

This condition is often linked with pregnancy, but it can also appear in men and women who aren't pregnant (usually over the age of 40). It usually consists of large patches of discoloration on the face and cheeks, often on the high points of the face like the cheeks, bridge of the nose, forehead and upper lip. It can be caused by hormone treatments, medication, sun exposure and pregnancy and is prevalent in women of color.

Melasma should be treated gently and carefully in skin of color. *Hydroquinone* is regularly recommended but this needs to be used extremely carefully with darker skin and isn't always the best option as it can cause unwanted effects on the skin (and can even make it darker). I think you know how I feel about **Hydro-quinone**, so I strongly advise if this option must be considered, to use it under strict doctor's guidance.

Pityriasis Alba

Pityriasis alba mostly affects children with darker skin on their face and arms but it has been known to appear on other areas of the body. In this instance, scaly patches of skin that are round and light in color form.

Unlike other conditions like vitiligo, the color change is temporary and disappears after treatment has been applied. This would usually need a medical diagnosis and medical treatment.

Pseudo Folliculitis (aka Razor Burn)

Because of the texture and coil of black hair, razor burn, ingrown hairs and bumps can be more prevalent in black skin.The hair can curl back on itself underneath the skin and cause an ingrown hair. This can lead to discomfort, infection and later, discoloration and hyperpigmentation.

It's a common side effect of shaving, so it may be recommended to try a different hair removal method that's more suitable for their skin. If infection is severe then this could present a contraindication. Otherwise, extraction of ingrown hairs may be needed to keep your client's skin healthy.

Vitiligo

Signs of vitiligo usually present themselves before adulthood. People with vitiligo have the same number of melanocytes (the cells that produce melanin and contribute to your skin tone) but they aren't active. This leads to patches of paler skin.

The condition is more noticeable in skin of color and is considered to be an autoimmune condition. This condition needs treatment from a skin specialist, but shouldn't present a contraindication to skin care treatments.

SKIN CONDITIONS THAT NEED TREATED DIFFERENTLY IN DARKER SKIN

There are some skin conditions that aren't necessarily more prevalent in darker skin, but need to be handled differently to lighter skin tones. Take the time to educate yourself further on how to handle these situations in all skin phototypes in addition to the overview provided here.

Here's a short overview of common skin conditions that may present differently, or need different treatment then identified in darker skin tones:

Acne

We all know what acne is, and know the impact that it can have on a clients self-esteem, wellbeing, health and comfort. It's likely that you'll recognise acne on darker skin - it sometimes comes with less nodules and cysts when it's present in darker skin, than in lighter skin - but what you need to be aware of is scarring.

Inflammation and skin wounds are big problems for dark skin when it comes to scarring and hyperpigmentation. Sometimes, even after acne has healed, the dark spots it leaves behind can be more visible than the acne was in the first place.

It's important to be gentle with acne-prone skin, but this is even more important with dark skin to prevent scarring. If you can reduce inflammation then this is important too.

Treat dark spots and patches caused by acne in the same way as hyperpigmentation (but please go carefully).

Contact Dermatitis

This usually displays as an itchy or burning rash. It's caused by contact with chemicals, heat or substances that a person is allergic to. It's basically a skin reaction. For darker skin this can lead to inflammation, hyper-pigmentation and skin damage. It may also look slightly different on darker skin in comparison to lighter skin.

Someone presenting with contact dermatitis needs medical care in order to deal with the reaction. Adding extra products, pressure or overhandling the skin could actually make the problem worse, so it's usually considered to be a contraindication.

Dry Skin

Dry skin can look a little different on darker skin. It may look dull, flaky, dry and lighter (also known as ashy skin). It's more common in areas like the knees or elbows, but can affect any area of the skin.

In darker skin, the skin's natural barrier can be more prone to water loss (due to having less ceramides in the skin) which can make it feel rough or dry. This may mean treating the skin with a rebalancing regimen to get it back in check and repair a damaged skin barrier.

Inflammation

Skin inflammation is a sign of an immune response in the body. Symptoms can include redness, heat, itching, sensitivity, and swelling. The cause or trigger of skin inflammation may be acute, such as a skin infection, or chronic, such as an autoimmune condition like psoriasis. It can also be caused by heat, skin damage or irritation.

Hypertension (high blood pressure) tends to be more prevalent in the black community in particular. This leads to swelling and water retention.

Inflammation and swelling can be seriously bad news for darker skin. It's a key cause of hyperpigmentation, caused by excess melanin production.

Psoriasis

Psoriasis is an autoimmune condition that causes inflammation as well as dry, red, itchy and scaly skin. It's usually pretty easy to spot on lighter but on darker skin, will appear as more purple patches with gray scales. On dark skin, the psoriasis patches may be more widespread, which can make it difficult to tell if you aren't familiar with it.

Active psoriasis usually needs to be managed medically, and any open sores or cracks will be a contraindication for skin treatments.

Rosacea

Rosacea is an auto-inflammatory skin condition. It has a range of different "levels" or some call it "grades" and over time is becoming more common in darker skin tones. It's easily missed on black skin by both medical professionals and people with the condition, as it was thought that darker skins don't experience rosacea. It turns out it's another case where it's been less familiar so has been missed.

Rosacea presents differently on darker skin than lighter skin. If a client with dark skin mentions that their face feels warm or flushed, burns or stings, discolors, has dry patches that appear swollen or has acne-type spots that don't clear up with treatment then it's worth referring them to seek a medical diagnosis of rosacea.

Seborrheic Dermatitis

This is an inflammatory skin condition that usually causes red, scaly patches on the scalp. It's an autoimmune disorder that can't be cured. The patches may also appear on the face and upper part of the body. Skin and hair products that contain alcohol can make it worse, and skin is usually sensitized so this is usually a treatment contraindication if it appears in an area you're going to be working on.

WORKING WITH DARKER SKIN (AS A PROFESSIONAL)

As you can see from the skin conditions above, your clients with dark skin will experience many of the same skin conditions as your light skinned clients. They'll experience some more often than those with lighter skin, and vice versa. There are also some skin conditions that you'll probably only see in skin that contains a higher level of melanin.

I cannot emphasize the importance of education on this topic enough. It's an absolutely essential part of the skin health equity process, and is how I believe we continue to develop skin health equity into our practice as skin care professionals.

One of the most important ways that you can practice, develop and grow your skin health equity approach is through knowledge. We all learn and gain new experiences every single day. If there was a hot new treatment out that everyone wanted a piece of, you'd level up and learn it.

As I've said before, my approach to skin health equity is *never* just about paying lip service to gain clients and make more money, but that's the reality. When I shout about the inequity in the beauty industry and how we can drive change - I mean it! However, it's also true that practicing skin health equity, being knowledgeable about *all* skin phototypes and working safely on a range of different types of skin can open up your doors to a much bigger customer base. It also enhances your reputation as a true professional, which can in turn bring more opportunities to your door.

It's also a kinder, inclusive and more human way to do business. In my opinion, those are business goals to strive for that are *just* as important as what's on your balance sheet.

When you're working with darker skin, whatever skin type, condition or shade that skin is, there are a few basics that are absolutely essential to bear in mind. If I'm being really honest, these should be the rules you should be sticking to whatever skin tone you're treating, not just darker skin tones.

Here are the main things you should be aware of when it comes to treating darker skin tones.

Avoid Causing Inflammation

Inflammation is the underrated enemy of darker skin, especially when it comes to hyperpigmentation and dark spots. Post-Inflammatory Hyperpigmentation (PIH) is caused by (you guessed it) inflammation.

Whether that's caused by a vigorous skin care treatment (like extractions, removals, piercing the skin, using needles), a heavy-handed massage, sun or heat damage, chemical burns or peels, product sensitivity or reactive skin conditions like acne, dermatitis or a skin infection - the results are the same. Boom, dark patches.

This can be even more distressing for the client if they have come to you for help with their pigmentation issues in the first place.

I believe that this sensitivity to inflammation is where the reputation that dark skin is "difficult" to deal with comes from. It's not that difficult! As a professional, you just need to understand that avoiding inflammation is in your clients' best interest - probably many of your clients, not just those with darker skin.

Skip The Skin Damage

I'm pretty sure that I don't have to over-explain this one (and if I do then we may need to take a step back and look at the bigger picture because something's not quite lining up here).

Skin damage is bad news for all skin phototypes, skin types and skin conditions.

Ok, there are some treatments that "damage" the skin in order to encourage healing and renewal like microneedling, laser and skin peels but guess what... these aren't always suitable for darker skin, or sensitive skin of any color.

With darker skin, skin damage can lead to hyperpigmentation, as I've already hammered home a couple of times now. It can also result in scarring (including keloid scarring), a damaged skin barrier and costly, time-consuming treatments to restore and repair. It also results in a lost customer that is extremely unlikely to recommend you (probably quite the opposite, let's be real) and struggles to feel confident with professionals in the industry.

Remember the survey back in chapter 2, where 92% of skin professionals suggested that they had seen skin damage on the clients as a result of improper use of technology? Never mind the more manual, hands-on side of the industry. It's a pretty shocking statistic, and though sadly it wasn't a surprise, that's almost every single skin pro who has had to deal with the negative effects caused by another in the industry.

It all boils down to a lack of ongoing education and training, and it's really the clients that suffer as a result. This in turn hurts the industry. I'll say it again: education is key.

Watch Those Products, Ingredients and Tools

Some products, ingredients and tools that are commonly used in skincare just aren't suitable for every type of skin for the reasons I've already outlined around inflammation and damage. There's a whole lot of misinformation out there.

Even some ingredients that I regularly see recommended as being great for darker skin...aren't so great.

If you do any research into hyperpigmentation, for example, *Hydroquinone* will come up as a solution time and time again. But actually, *Hydroquinone* needs to be used with *extreme* caution on darker skin. It can cause damage or even contact dermatitis, which in turn can turn into even darker hyperpigmentation. If it isn't used correctly, it can leave a lighter 'halo' effect around the area that was treated, leaving it even more pronounced and noticeable.

Ingredients and products that are irritating, harsh or strip the skin of its natural balance - such as overly drying *SD Alcohols* or rough physical exfoliators - can damage the skin. Even chemical exfoliators that are routinely used in 'safe' concentrations may be too much for dark skin.

In general, you want to steer clear of anything that's going to cause irritation to the skin or cause inflammation. This is a good rule of thumb for every type of skin out there. Here's what to avoid:

- Overly fragranced skin care.
- Abrasive scrubs and facial cleansing brushes with stiff bristles.
- Bar soaps.
- Irritating ingredients such as *Menthol, Mint, Eucalyptus, Lemon* or *SD/Denatured Alcohol.*
- High percentage acids.
- High concentrations of *Hydroquinone.*
- Some types of laser, peels and microneedling treatments.

Focus on gentle, nourishing skin care that isn't going to cause breakouts, damage, inflammation or irritation to the skin. For instance, you can still achieve great results with more frequent peels that are less invasive.

I would be remiss, if I did not talk about some great ingredients to use instead of *Hydroquinone* to target pigmentation concerns and concerns leading to hyperpigmentation. This is not an exhaustive list, but in my opinion, these are extremely supportive ingredients to treating hyperpigmentation, without compromising the skin's integrity:

- *Lactic Acid* naturally possesses a lower pH,

making it a more effective Acid without higher concentrations. It also is a great Tyrosine inhibitor and it also brightens and hydrates.

- *Glycolic Acid* in lower concentrations can still be highly effective, targeting aging and loss of tone.
- *Salicylic Acid* is a very effective anti-inflammatory and antibacterial Acid, helping to prevent hyper-pigmentation.
- Honourable mentions to *Azelaic Acid, Mandelic Acid, Rosehip Extract, Vitamin A* derivatives, *Vitamin C, Bromelain* and *Papain*.

Did I mention that education is key? By this I mean both education for you as a professional and your own professional responsibility to educate your clients on how to take care of their skin. I get it, I won't seem to let this go, but it's the truth.

SKIN THEOLOGIAN'S TIP

When it comes to education, think inclusive. Look for training and education programs where you will have the opportunity to learn about - and work on - all types of skin. This is essential for skin health equity.

Things are definitely improving when it comes to education. Many training providers, educators and schools are committing to offering a diverse range of experience, voices and training opportunities.

If you're an educator (or an aspiring one) then it's up to you to provide these opportunities to the next generation of skin professionals. Think about skin health equity and encouraging discovery in everything you do.

HOW TO HAVE CQ CONVERSATIONS ABOUT SKIN CONDITIONS WITH CLIENTS

Many of the points I've already made about CQ conversations still stand in this chapter, but when it comes to skin conditions, there are a few points I want to make about skin condition conversations with your clients who have darker skin, especially if you're from a different cultural background.

Here are the points to understand when it comes to speaking with CQ:

- Don't make assumptions - using professional expertise and your skin pro powers of deduction is one thing, making an assumption that "every person with darker skin tones has this, that's all it could possibly be", without a proper investigation isn't how to do it.

- Ask the right questions and ask them in a sensitive way, particularly around topics that might make someone feel uncomfortable or "othered".

- Do your research, so that you're prepared for questions and conversations with your clients about their skin. No one wants to hear "well I've never seen that before" or hear that you have no idea what to do with their skin. A picture paints a thousand words, so brush up on what common skin conditions look like on all different types of skin.

- This should go without saying but be sensitive about contraindications, even if you've never seen a particular presentation before. If you can't treat someone because their condition might leave their skin open to harm, discomfort or infection then they need to know that. But you can communicate that in a culturally sensitive and appropriate manner that comes from a place of care, not a brush-off.

- Listen to your client but exercise your professional judgment. They will know their skin and how it makes them feel. However, as a pro you know what's actually safe and what's best for their skin from a science and reactive perspective. Don't be pushed into treatments that are unsafe, unhelpful or damaging for the client just because you don't want to offend them or you're worried about how to tell them it's not safe - that's part of managing their wellbeing as a professional. Remember to communicate this in a sensible and sensitive way.

If you're professional and knowledgeable in your conversations with clients with darker skin about what they need for their routine and ongoing treatments, they will **trust** you to handle their skin with care. Let your results do the talking, and your education and expertise shine through. It might not be an overnight process as you're working to undo a lot of mistrust and unease from people who may have been let down in the past.

KEY TAKEAWAYS

- Darker skin experiences the same issues as lighter skin, but it may appear differently on the skin, so it's important to recognise it.

- There are some skin conditions that are more prevalent in darker skin.
- Sometimes darker skin needs to be treated differently, and it's important that this is done sensitively without 'othering'.

6

MANUAL LYMPHATIC DRAINAGE (MLD) FOR DARKER SKIN

*J*n this chapter, you'll learn about:

- What MLD is.
- The Benefits of MLD as A Pro Treatment.
- Why MLD is great for hyperpigmentation.
- MLD Tips.
- What To Avoid With MLD.

WHAT IS MANUAL LYMPHATIC DRAINAGE (MLD)?

Let's start with the lymphatic system and what it does. You may already know this, but I want to start at the beginning. The lymphatic system works to keep body fluids in balance and to keep the body's natural defenses up. It's made up of a network of vessels that carry lymph throughout the body, from your head to your body. Lymph is a clear, watery fluid that contains proteins, salts and other substances, like white blood cells known as lymphocytes. The lymphatic system gets rid of cell waste and acts as a one-way drainage system - but unlike other systems in the body, such as blood circulation, it doesn't have its own pumping mechanism.

Sometimes, the lymphatic system doesn't quite work as it should. Medical treatment, illness, skin disorders, stress, insomnia, fatigue and even migraines can all stop your lymphatic system from functioning correctly. This can lead to swelling and inflammation, or even medical conditions like lymphedema.

Manual Lymphatic Drainage (MLD) can help improve circulation and reduce inflammation and swelling. It's a non-invasive treatment that can work well with other steps like exercise, compression garments and skincare routines. It can be carried out on the whole body, selected areas or even just the face.

In my professional opinion, the fact that it reduces inflammation and swelling without being an invasive procedure, or breaking the skin makes it great for darker skin tones. It doesn't damage the skin *and* it reduces inflammation.

It can be a safer option than other processes to rejuve-nate and lift the skin when it comes to skin of color. When I talk about having alternative options available rather than just turning darker skinned potential clients away, this is the type of thing that I mean. It can be extremely effective without the risks that come with certain other treatments for melanin-rich skin.

At-home MLD has been growing in popularity over recent years as people explore treatments that they can try at home like gua sha and face yoga. This is likely as a result of the pandemic causing everyone to take more care of their health and wellness, as well as their skin. They've also had more time on their hands (quite liter-ally) to explore new routines.

Gua sha uses a small tool to massage the skin's surface, improving circulation, contouring the face and supporting draining. Face yoga works on similar prin-ciples, but with a focus on facial exercises and manip-ulation.

Both are used for anti-aging benefits, improving circu-lation and improving the appearance of the skin. Whilst it's important to get a little self-care in as often as you can, there are some risks with a DIY approach. The wrong pressure or technique can be used, with no-one around to correct it. Even an unawareness of the lymphatic system's map on the face and body can lead to incorrect flow and direction of lymph, which gives the wrong results. A lack of hygiene or using the wrong products can happen too.

At best, it renders the session ineffective but at worst an individual could actually be damaging their skin.

PROFESSIONAL MLD TREATMENTS

We can jump straight into the benefits of a professional MLD treatment for your client, and how to frame it as a treatment:

- Can help to fight off infection.
- May help speed up healing and recovery from the cold and flu.
- Reduce water retention.
- Improve cellulite, skin swelling, scar tissue, acne, and stretch marks.
- Reduce stress and fatigue.
- Help with post-exercise recovery.
- Can help to reduce signs of aging.
- Reduces puffy skin and inflammation, therefore preventing potential hyperpigmentation.
- Can sculpt and tone the face by smoothing out the connective tissue in the face.
- Encourages circulation.
- Brightens and adds radiance to the skin.

In addition, It can also be used to help individuals suffering from health concerns such as insomnia, fatigue and arthritis.

All of these benefits come from a non-invasive treatment that doesn't use any active products that could cause issues for darker skin (or skin of any shade). The other great option is that it can be incorporated into a facial or other skincare routines easily.

SKIN THEOLOGIAN'S TIP

Let's just pause to talk about inflammation and swelling. I've already highlighted that inflammation and swelling leads to hyperpigmentation, dark spots and damage in darker skin.

One thing it's also worth discussing is the fact that hypertension - a form of high blood pressure that causes swelling (especially in the ankles, feet and hands) is more prevalent in the black community. Studies have shown that black men and women are around 15% more likely to experience hypertension, particularly as they age.

If your darker skinned clients come to you with concerns around swelling, inflammation or blood pressure then this may be the cause. Of course, you need to ask this question in your consultation.

How To Carry Out A Facial MLD Treatment As A Pro

This isn't a training manual, and I'd always recommend that you seek additional resources and training ahead of carrying out MLD on a client.

A MLD massage is different to the usual types of facial massage that are usually carried out, but can still be just as relaxing and effective for reducing tension. It's important to understand those differences and be clear on how to carry the treatment out in the most effective way that helps your clients to get results.

You don't need any special tools

Massaging with your hands is absolutely fine, and can help you to tune into the clients skin, their feelings and the massage process itself.

Make circular movements toward lymph nodes

In order to drain lymphatic fluid, massage the face with the pads of your fingers, always working upward and from the middle of the face toward the lymph nodes around the neck and ears. The key to a good MLD massage is to use gentle movements. It's important to apply very light pressure to stimulate tissues, not necessarily blood flow, as the lymph vessels are just below the skin. I usually repeat each step six times for best results.

Massage without oil or cream

To optimize drainage, this should be a "dry" massage, i.e., without applying oils or creams to the skin. So, if you want to incorporate MLD into your client's skincare routine, start by cleansing their face, then perform your massage before applying any further skincare products. You can then move onto the rest of the facial treatment, if that's part of the procedure your client has booked.

If you do need to incorporate a product into your MLD protocol, for example if your client has very dry skin, I'd recommend nothing beyond a light essence.

Use upward and outward motions

The golden rule with MLD is to always work upward and outward when massaging. Start with the neck, then move up to the jawline and chin, gradually work up to the mouth, nose, eyes, and glabella (the space between the eyebrows), and finish by massaging the forehead.

Make it a regular thing

As with most skincare treatments, MLD gives the best results when it's carried out regularly. A one-off session is likely to only give short term results.

I have seen *significant* improvement in hyperpigmentation rates when MLD has been incorporated alongside the right treatments and home care routines.

Aftercare

As with all treatments, aftercare is an important part of MLD. Again, take your time to train in this treatment, but generally to get the best results, you want to advise your clients to do the following for at least 24 hours after treatment:

- Loosen tight clothing.
- Drinking plenty of water is recommended alongside lymphatic draining, to keep the body hydrated and to help clear the body.

- Reduce caffeine intake.
- Avoid alcohol for 24 hours.
- Cut down on smoking.
- Make time to rest and relax.
- Regular (but not too strenuous) exercise helps with muscle contraction, therefore lymph flow.
- Low sodium diets are recommended for a healthy lymphatic system – poor diets are a contributing factor to poor MLD.

SKIN THEOLOGIAN'S TIP

Did you know that the time of day can make a difference when it comes to MLD? A morning treatment is great for reducing inflammation and puffiness. It also helps to prep the skin for daytime skincare products.

An evening treatment (or one later in the day) can help with relaxation and de-stressing.

It's important to stay at the forefront of health and wellness trends within the industry so that you can continue to meet the needs of your clients. Keeping your skills up to date and learning how to do the treatments that your clients want is important. Never underestimate the power of tried and true treatments. And MLD is certainly a classic that I believe has been underused, especially for darker skin.

KEY TAKEAWAYS

- Staying aware of skincare trends and development is essential as a skin professional.
- MLD can be a great way to reduce inflammation and swelling.
- MLD is a non-invasive treatment that's safe and extremely beneficial for darker skin.

7

SKIN BLEACHING (AKA THE B-WORD)

*I*n this chapter, you'll learn about:

- The history of skin bleaching.
- A cultural perspective on skin bleaching.
- Why skin bleaching is bad for skin, health and mind.
- How to have those sensitive conversations with clients who may be bleaching their skin.

SKIN BLEACHING: AN INTRODUCTION

If you aren't from a cultural background where skin bleaching exists, then it might not be a familiar topic to you. It's deep-rooted and prevalent in certain cultures, often passed down within families. Many people start out bleaching their skin from a young age, encouraged by parents or seeing it set as an example.

We'll talk about the reasons for bleaching the skin, how it fits with culture and how to approach the topic sensitively and appropriately, with cultural intelligence.

Skin bleaching isn't just bad for skin health. It's bad for health overall, including mental health, self-esteem and confidence. It's a complex issue that's often deep-rooted in shame and worry.

I'll start with an example I saw recently at the grocery store. As I left my car and approached the front doors, I heard and saw three young, happy boys of color who were playing outside of the grocery store. They seemed to be brothers aged between 6-12 years old. One of the boys called out to their mother who was standing nearby in the shade (one thing to remember is that skin bleaching can make your skin extremely photo-sensitive - even without bleaching many people with darker skin are encourage to "stay out of the sun" so their skin doesn't become darker). As I looked at their mother, the first thing I noticed was that she was a beautiful black woman dressed in traditional African clothing. She looked like royalty.

The second thing I noticed made my heart sink.

Her skin tone was extremely pale, with an almost gray tint to it, very unlike the skin of her sons. Obviously genetics sometimes work in mysterious ways, and I didn't see their father, so perhaps that isn't relevant.

However, I noticed her knuckles were dark and that her skin looked tight and flat, with that conspicuous gray tone. A tone that isn't generally found naturally in skin of any color. Her skin was uniform in its lightness, which isn't usually the case with skin conditions like vitiligo or hyperpigmentation (the truth is everyone's skin and body is full of different skin tones). These are all signs of skin bleaching, and signs that she had probably been bleaching her skin for quite a number of years.

This was heartbreaking to me. This beautiful, regal woman had felt the need to put herself through discomfort and risk her health all for the sake of making her skin lighter. It got me thinking.

- What had made her feel that bleaching her skin this way was the right option?
- What message was this sending out to her sons?
- If this woman was my client, how would I approach this with her?
- How would that conversation happen if I was of a different ethnicity?

WHY DO PEOPLE BLEACH THEIR SKIN?

The short answer is that they want their skin to appear lighter. They equate darker skin with being less attractive than lighter skin.

They may have gotten this impression from their community, the media or from someone influential in their life (such as a family member or partner). For whatever reason they perceive that lighter skin is beautiful, perpetuating in the myths that have been set up culturally for hundreds of years.

Unfortunately colorism is prevalent within communities of color, particularly in some cultures where it's rooted in historical factors like colonialism. It's commonplace in many African countries, in the Caribbean, in India and in the Middle East - as well as countries where people from these countries have moved to over time, such as the US, Canada and the UK

It's a cultural and societal problem as much as it is an individual issue. For years, the media has pushed the agenda that "lighter is better". This pressure has also come from within the black community and from within families.

Skin bleaching may start out relatively innocently (if that's possible), with a view to lightening up dark patches of hyperpigmentation on the skin. It may start out completely intentionally in a quest for lighter skin. But it can soon descend into the type of all-over skin bleaching as I've mentioned earlier.

Skin bleaching isn't necessarily hidden either. Even in countries where the ingredients are banned, you will find bleaching agents for sale. In other countries, they're produced and marketed - by some of the largest health and beauty brands in the world - as a beauty aid. Bleaching products are openly advertised, sold on the shelves and available for purchase by anyone.

And people buy and use them, with little regard for their health. You may think it's niche and not something you need to worry about personally for your clients, but the reality is that millions of women are spending billions of dollars on skin bleaching products every year.

WHAT'S THE PROBLEM WITH SKIN BLEACHING?

The problems with skin bleaching aren't just skin deep. They go *much* further than that unfortunately; but let's start there since this is a skin care resource.

How Bleaching Affects The Skin

There are two types of ways that skin bleaching is carried out. There are the products that are bought (either under or over the counter) to lighten skin that contain ingredients to inhibit melanin production, destroy melanocytes (responsible for making melanin) or prevent melanin from being deposited into the skin.

The other type of bleaching products are the home-made kind. Yep, you read that correctly. Mixing up all sorts of caustic, dangerous concoctions at home that are designed to be applied directly to the skin.

Whichever method is used, it comes with risks and hazards for the skin. This ranges from rashes, discoloration (that gray tone I mentioned earlier), dry skin, dull skin, scarring, tightness, sensitivity through to a reduction in the overall health of your skin. It essentially destroys the skin's natural microbiome and natural defenses. It also leaves skin more sensitive to the sun and can open up the risk of serious skin issues, such as skin cancer.

Skin bleaching weakens the skin and leaves it more prone to premature aging. Some ingredients cause broken veins or thinner skin over time. They can also leave skin more susceptible to visible bruising.

The other reality is that it leaves skin looking unnatural in terms of color, texture and tone. There's no richness or warmth to bleached skin and it often looks dry, tight and dull - that's usually the easiest way to recognise skin that's been subjected to bleach.

I've previously discussed ingredients to go easy on when it comes to skincare for darker skin tones. The main goals are to avoid irritation, inflammation and damage as this leads to pigmentation issues. Well, the ingredients in skin bleaching agents (SBAs) can do all of the above, and can actually contribute to skin damage in this way.

How Bleaching Affects Physical Health

Skin bleaching doesn't just stop at skin damage. The chemicals used in bleaching can cause breathing issues, eye problems, liver and kidney damage, neurological problems, cancer and stillbirths. Plus, because with some homemade bleaching creations, you never quite know what's in it so establishing the true damage caused by it is something of an unknown.

Certain skin bleaching agents (SBAs) can cause a whole host of problems with physical health. They can damage the nervous system, accumulate in the body and even contribute to health issues linked to blood pressure, osteoporosis and weight gain. Other ingredients contribute to thyroid problems.

The World Health Organization (WHO) has issued a statement that skin bleaching should be treated as a public health concern, as it's so prevalent and so damaging.

How Bleaching Affects Mental Health

There are so many studies now to show how early young children become aware of their appearance and the societal pressures to fit in. The mental impact of this is startling. Skin bleaching and societal beauty standards - including the myth that lighter is better - go hand in hand with this.

If you are constantly being told that your skin is too dark, and taking risks like rubbing caustic chemicals onto your skin, that suggests a certain level of mental impact on your wellbeing. If the pressure is coming from your family or loved ones, then that can create issues around not feeling like you're enough or that you're loved in the skin you're in.

It creates insecurity, unhappiness and constantly links your body image with a place of negativity. If you stop bleaching your skin, your melanin may or may not come back. If someone is in the headspace that they aren't beautiful with darker skin, this quickly becomes a cycle of shame, worry, skin bleaching and negative thinking.

It's extremely complex, but extremely important to understand that it's not "just" skin lightening. It comes from hundreds of years of history, pressure and beauty standards that weren't created with melanin-rich skin in mind.

Contraindications Caused By Skin Bleaching

Skin bleaching isn't just a problem for your client. It's potentially a problem for you as a skin professional too. Skin bleaching can, and usually will, compromise the skin in one way or another. You definitely have to be aware of some contraindications that arise when clients have lightened their skin in some way or another.

I'll take you through how you can have those culturally sensitive conversations with your clients around skin bleaching later on in the chapter, but let's focus on the treatment aspect for now. We'll talk about *how* skin bleaching agents (SBAs) work in the next section so that you can understand what you're dealing with in a little more detail. I'd recommend speaking to your suppliers or educating yourself in more detail on this topic.

As skin is compromised and/or traumatized after skin bleaching, you should avoid recommending (or using) acids, exfoliants or peels. You can be honest with the client and tell them that their skin isn't in the right condition for these treatments. Skin should be recovered, healed and strengthened before you use any of these treatments, so it may be better to focus on those aspects and to let the client know that this is what you're doing and why.

The other reality is that you - and often, the client - have no idea what they've been putting on their skin. They just know they want it to be lighter and that it seems to be working. This can be a real challenge as a professional as it becomes difficult to know how skin will react or how products will react to the products already used on their skin. A thorough cleanse should always be part of the treatment.

HOW DOES SKIN BLEACHING WORK?

Let's get technical. Skin bleaching for darker skin tones aims to reduce, inhibit production of or remove melanin from the skin. You'll remember that melanin is what's responsible for the color of darker skin (and gives additional benefits like slightly more sun protection which leads to reduced visible signs of aging - your darker skinned clients absolutely need to wear sunscreen).

Mostly, skin bleaching agents (SBAs) are used topically and often come as a cream or a lotion. They're applied to the skin, focusing on the areas of "concern". This often eventually becomes the whole body. There are also skin lightening tablets and shots on the market that interfere with the body's natural melanin production, though there's very little scientific evidence to support that these actually work.

Here's how many of the main skin bleaching agents (SBAs) work on the natural melanin in skin to lighten the skin:

- They inhibit the activity of an enzyme called Tyrosinase. This enzyme is what the body converts into melanin so by holding it back the idea is that it pauses melanin production too.
- They prevent melanin from being deposited onto the skin from the melanocyte cells to the surrounding keratinocyte cells (this is a natural function). Some processes stop melanin from getting from the body to the surface of your skin. Over time the melanin is not replaced.
- By destroying the melanin and melanocytes in the skin to stop melanin production.

There is a big difference between influencing the skin to be at its best and *stopping* your skin from functioning in a way that is normal and correct. Healthy skin should be allowed to thrive in its natural form.

Hydroquinone and *Mercury* are commonly used to lighten the skin. It goes without saying that *Mercury* is extremely toxic and bad for your health, causing serious health issues. *Hydroquinone*, though commonly used in small amounts in skincare, isn't good for the skin when used in large amounts and over a long period of time.

Anything that is actively destroying key parts of the skin's structure (such as melanin) or production isn't necessarily a good thing. Especially when it's unregulated, unmonitored and unchecked.

TALKING ABOUT SKIN BLEACHING WITH YOUR CLIENTS (WITH CQ)

As with any conversation with your clients, it's important to show empathy and never to judge. We always want to ensure we're educating and informing clients, never passing judgment or feeling like we're dictating to them.

If you are from a different cultural background to your client - and one that doesn't have a history of skin bleaching ingrained into it - then this adds another dimension to the conversation. One of cultural intelligence, where the client is not left feeling patronized, offended or feeling like "well what would you know about it?" As I mentioned earlier, the cultural issues around skin lightening and bleaching are complex, to say the least.

In this situation, it becomes even more important to educate yourself and to act with CQ. Never assume, and never write it off as "just part of culture". It may well be, but that doesn't mean that it's right - that also doesn't mean that it's necessarily your place to judge it in that way.

If all the signs are pointing towards the fact that a client is bleaching their skin, it's a topic to approach with kindness and professionalism. The reality is, you only need to know what's going on from a skin care perspective. It isn't your job to judge - sadly, it's probably so ingrained that they may not listen to someone from outside their culture.

Remember, you're looking for gray-tinged skin that appears dull and tight, discrepancies in other areas of the skin, dryness and thin skin.

SKIN THEOLOGIAN'S TIP

Remember, there are some skin conditions and concerns that cause the skin to lighten or appear lighter. These include issues such as vitiligo, albinism, scarring and other conditions that may usually look red on lighter skin, but appear differently on darker skin. These skin conditions won't usually have the gray-blue hue that comes with skin bleaching.

Your client may already be self conscious about these changes to their natural pigmentation (or lack of pigmentation when it comes to albinism). Ask any questions - that are relevant to the treatment - sensitively and carefully. Don't just jump straight into a conversation about skin bleaching. I wouldn't recommend this even if your client is fairly obviously bleaching their skin.

Here are some questions to consider including in your consultation if you feel that your client is using bleaching agents on their skin:

- Can you tell me about how your skin has been feeling lately?

- How do you feel about your skin health overall?
- If you could address one thing about your skin, what would that one thing be"? (This may have the client draw attention to related side effects like tightness, lack of radiance, dullness and increased sensitivity).
- The normal medication questionnaire -should also include "Are you currently or have you used any topical 'lightening, bleaching or pigment altering creams or skin lightening agents in the last 12 months"? (Give the client a chance to answer themselves on this matter.)
- Do you have any medical conditions that affect your skin? This can be useful for identifying other skin conditions that may be confused with bleached skin.
- Have you always worn SPF? Or can you tell me when you started wearing SPF?
- Please list the primary reasons for your SPF skin habits?

You don't need to call them out or confront them, even if you're 99% sure that they're bleaching their skin and they tell you they're not. It's important to treat the client with respect and honor. If they've chosen not to disclose this to you, it's not your role as a professional to shame, judge or upset them about this. Remember, skin, health and culture often goes hand-in-hand and is long-standing. It's a complicated subject that's often steeped in external and internal influences. It's unlikely that you'll change their mind on the topic.

If a client has been open with you and disclosed that they're using skin bleaching agents (SBAs) on their skin, try and find out what they're using. Even if they can take a photo of the product, bring it in or Google it for you. This obviously won't work if they're using something homemade, but it's important to be armed with as much information as possible. If they're ready to talk, be ready to listen.

If you feel that a client is open to a discussion about skin bleaching, or that they're remorseful about bleaching their skin, then this may be the time to explain some of the risks. Keep it impersonal, factual and friendly. Don't dictate or judge. They may not come away from the session ready to put down the bleach for good, but they may remember a professional that took the time to educate them with kindness when they needed it. They may then be in a position to go away and do some more research on the topic. The reality is that bleaching may have been so normalized in their household that they may not realize just how dangerous and unhealthy it can be.

For skin that seems as if it is being bleached, or where the client has confirmed that this is the case, it needs to be treated gently, as you would any compromised skin that's lacking in balance. Treat any skin concerns that they identify (or that you identify) such as sensitivity, tightness or thinning skin.

Use comforting products and avoid anything that could sensitize their skin further. Focus on healing, recovering and strengthening skin rather than using active ingredients like acids, exfoliants or peels.

Be open with the client about why you're taking this approach. You don't need to say "I'm doing this because you're bleaching your skin and lying about it", but do say something like "I've noticed your skin is dry and tight so I've used these products to rebalance, comfort and nourish the skin."

It's likely that the client already has some insecurities around their skin, and they may have concerns about their appearance. It might have taken them completely out of their comfort zone to visit you. Being critical or judgmental is never helpful in this situation, even if you're a "tough love" kind of professional.

SKIN BLEACHING: A FINAL WORD

I think I've probably made my thoughts on skin bleaching and lightening relatively clear in this chapter. I have had clients who have bleached their skin in the past and clients who have constantly had skin bleaching pushed on them by family as an option, suggestion and recommendation. I've never judged them for those decisions, but I've worked with them on solutions.

It's tough, and it can be a tough conversation to have. I imagine even more so when you're outside of that particular community and have no experience of attitudes towards skin lightening and the perception that lighter skin is a "goal" and beauty standard to reach for.

This isn't true. Black and brown skin is absolutely beautiful in its natural form. There's no need to create gray, damaged skin. But it's a personal choice for your clients to make.

KEY TAKEAWAYS

- Skin bleaching is bad for the skin. There's no other way to say it.
- It's often a cultural issue so needs to be approached and discussed with real care.

- Remove any judgment from the situation and leave the door open for a conversation with your client.

8

TEN COMMANDMENTS FOR SKIN PROFESSIONALS TO PRACTICE SKIN HEALTH EQUITY AND CQ

1. Treat your clients equally but be mindful of differences

This is the overarching concept behind CQ and acting as a compassionate and understanding skin professional. It's being able to have sensitive conversations, utilize your professional expertise and adjust your treatments wherever it's necessary. It's being open to discussion and open to new ideas or experiences that are different to yours.

2. Never make assumptions

Unless it's something that falls in the realms of your professional expertise, don't make assumptions, especially when it comes to the culture of others. Even if you feel it comes from a positive place, that may not come across as intended.

3. Keep your education up to date

This is important as a skin professional overall, and is even more important when it comes to different skin phototypes. Thankfully education is changing in a positive way to incorporate a comprehensive range of skin and hair types. There's still a way to go, and we as professionals are the ones who can make the change.

4. Be culturally sensitive

If you need to make adjustments for treatments, or show empathy and understanding in a situation that is different to your own culture and background then do it with sensitivity and kindness.

5. Be aware when it comes to products, treatments and tools

Level up your knowledge on the tools, treatments and products that work for every type of skin out there. You need to understand these to be able to treat your clients effectively, safely and with care. It's part of your commitment to being a skin professional.

6. Using The Right Laser For Darker Skin Is Important

The commandment says it all. Recommending and carrying out laser treatments on dark skin should be researched and proven to be ideal for darker skin. Not all lasers are created equally. Understanding the differences is significantly important to a safe and results oriented service for melanin-rich skin. Take the time to do a thorough consultation and to offer other options in the interests of true skin health equity.

7. Create treatments, training and client spaces with CQ in mind

Embed CQ into every part of your role as a skin professional. Whether you're a business owner, a contractor, educator, or you have another part to play in the industry - we all need to do whatever we can to make a difference.

8. Be aware of skin bleaching

You may not be familiar with it, you may not truly understand the reasons behind it and you may not have been trained to spot it. Educate yourself on the topic and how to work with skin that's been bleached. But never judge and always keep the conversation sensitive. It's the client's choice if they want to disclose it - you can treat their skin concerns as they are right now.

9. The Fitzpatrick Scale isn't the best measure of skin photo type

It's too broad, not inclusive and doesn't serve its purpose. It's overused and underwhelming. The good news is that alternatives are on the way from some of the biggest tech and research groups in the world. I personally cannot wait.

10. We're all human.

That's the theme that underpins this entire book, and the entire concept of CQ. Your clients may have different reasons for visiting you in a professional capacity, but the overarching theme is that everyone wants to look and feel good, whatever their background.

Conclusion

Ok, we've covered a lot in this book.

You've taken the time to read this book and grow your understanding of inclusion, CQ and skin health equality as an industry professional. You have the ability to drive change and make it a better environment for skin professionals and clients alike.

For far too long, the beauty industry has not had diverse representation on the agenda, which has led to a lack of trust, knowledge and understanding. This has allowed inaccurate information to flourish in both a professional and client capacity.

The biggest feedback I hear from skin professionals is that they don't always feel comfortable having conversations. They feel that they don't know where the line is between professional advice and conversations that may seem insensitive. This isn't just a problem within the beauty industry.

CQ is here to stay. We need to embrace it and empower our colleagues, peers, students, clients and industry leaders to operate within its parameters. We need to celebrate the diversity within our client base and within our teams, and we need to utilize the range of knowledge and experiences that come with this diversity to enable everyone to thrive.

We can all do better. And I firmly believe that it starts with education. From the beginning, training needs to cover every type of skin and hair that a professional may need to treat. Ongoing training, brand updates and short courses all need to embed skin health equity and diversity. Skin care educators need to provide opportunities for their students to work on a range of different skin types and photo types so that they can get real hands-on experience that they can take forward in their career.

Your clients need to be educated too. Whether it's about understanding their own melanin-rich skin and dispelling some of the myths and misconceptions that they've absorbed over time. It will be no surprise to you that many clients don't understand their own skin. As a skin professional, you should certainly be a part of that journey of growth, education and understanding.

The No Compromise Black Skin Care Guide: The Truth About Caring For Darker Skin Volume I was the first book I created, to educate skin enthusiasts with darker skin about darker skin and how to take care of it. It existed as a resource to help counter some of the terrible advice that I have seen those in the black community end up on the receiving end of. The type of bad advice that leads to long-term skin damage that takes time, patience and significant effort to resolve. This then perpetuates the cycle of mistrust and misinformation that is far too prevalent for those with darker skin.

If your clients are looking for a resource to help them to better understand their skin then I would recommend they start there, with Volume 1. It's a no-nonsense, practical guide to caring for darker skin that aims to empower them to choose the right products, professionals and treatments . Even as an industry professional, it's likely that you will learn something from this book also, though it's written in a way that speaks directly to the consumer. There are industry insights throughout, and research from skin professionals.

The response to the first book was overwhelming and it's ultimately what led to me writing this book. The onus shouldn't just be on clients to understand their skin. Those in the industry need to understand it too.

They also need to be able to have sensitive conversations with their clients that come from a place of empathy and understanding. CQ and skin health equity have been on my radar for a *long* time, but this doesn't always translate across the wider industry. I think this is one of the most important cultural shifts that can happen to the community of skin professionals.

Progress *is* being made. Over the last few years in particular, the beauty industry (and the industries around it) have talked a good talk. And in some cases, they've turned that talk into action. They're improving their understanding of a range of skin phototypes, they're making their marketing material more reflective of their diverse audience, they're hiring talent from different backgrounds and they're creating more inclusive products.

New brands have launched that cater to a wider range of skin tones. Other brands have been launched by founders of color. The conversation is starting to feel more inclusive, and no longer treating those with darker skin tones as 'others' or an afterthought.

Even the tech industry - which has been aligned with the beauty industry since the beginning - has recognized this, developing technological solutions to traditional tools that are letting people of color down. This is the type of innovation that happens once an industry starts to listen to a diverse range of experiences, perspectives and backgrounds.

It's essential that this progress doesn't lose momentum. Inclusion, skin healthy equity and CQ are not trends. They are industry transformers that act as catalysts for welcomed and innovative growth for one of the most brilliant industries there is: BEAUTY.

C. R. Cooper
The Skin Theologian

I'd love to stay connected with you beyond this resource. I hope you do too.

C.R.COOPER

THE SKIN THEOLOGIAN

Connect with me on IG at:
@theskintheologian

and/or connect at
www.skintheologian.com
for additional resources and updates.

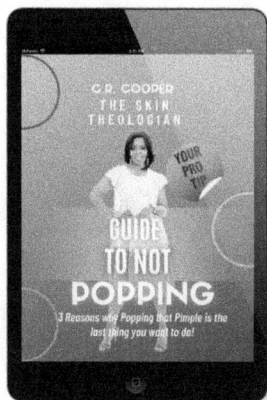

References

Skin color in dermatology textbooks: An updated evaluation and analysis

https://www.jaad.org/article/S0190-9622(20)30700-3/fulltext

Dermatology lacks diversity

https://www.mdedge.com/dermatology/article/108920/practice-management/dermatology-lacks-diversity#:~:text=Today%2C%20black%20dermatologists%20comprise%203,3%5D%3A584-7

Dermatologic Health Disparities

https://www.ncbi.nlm.nih.gov/pmc/articles/PMC3742002/

Study finds gender and skin-type bias in commercial artificial-intelligence systems

https://news.mit.edu/2018/study-finds-gender-skin-type-bias-artificial-intelligence-systems-0212

Black Impact: Consumer Categories Where African Americans Move Markets

https://www.nielsen.com/us/en/insights/article/2018/black-impact-consumer-categories-where-african-americans-move-markets/

Melanoma Among Non-Hispanic Black Americans

https://www.cdc.gov/pcd/issues/2019/18_0640.htm

2020 Plastic Surgery Statistics | Procedures by Ethnicity

https://www.plasticsurgery.org/documents/News/Statistics/2020/cosmetic-procedures-ethnicity-2020.pdf

Acral Lentiginous Melanoma

https://www.ncbi.nlm.nih.gov/books/NBK559113/

Skin Cancer Concerns in People of Color: Risk Factors and Prevention

https://www.ncbi.nlm.nih.gov/pmc/articles/PMC5454668/

Google searches for new measure of skin tones to curb bias in products

https://www.reuters.com/business/sustainable-business/exclusive-google-searches-new-measure-skin-tones-curb-bias-products-2021-06-18/

Racial Differences in Hypertension: Implications for High Blood Pressure Management

https://www.ncbi.nlm.nih.gov/pmc/articles/PMC4108512/

Mercury in skin lightening products

https://www.who.int/publications/i/item/WHO-CED-PHE-EPE-19.13

www.ingramcontent.com/pod-product-compliance
Lightning Source LLC
Chambersburg PA
CBHW070927030426
42336CB00014BA/2575